Head and Neck Pathology

Editor

JUSTIN A. BISHOP

SURGICAL PATHOLOGY CLINICS

www.surgpath.theclinics.com

Consulting Editor
JASON L. HORNICK

March 2021 • Volume 14 • Number 1

ELSEVIER

1600 John F. Kennedy Boulevard • Suite 1800 • Philadelphia, Pennsylvania, 19103-2899

http://www.theclinics.com

SURGICAL PATHOLOGY CLINICS Volume 14, Number 1
March 2021 ISSN 1875-9181, ISBN-13: 978-0-323-77630-1

Editor: Katerina Heidhausen
Developmental Editor: Donald Mumford

Surgical Pathology Clinics (ISSN 1875-9181) is published quarterly by Elsevier Inc., 360 Park Avenue South, New York, NY 10010. Months of issue are March, June, September, and December. Business and Editorial Office: Elsevier Inc., 1600 John F. Kennedy Blvd., Ste. 1800, Philadelphia, PA 19103-2899. Accounting and Circulation Offices: Elsevier Inc., 3251 Riverport Lane, Maryland Heights, MO 63043. Periodicals postage paid at New York, NY and at additional mailing offices. Subscription prices are $228.00 per year (US individuals), $358.00 per year (US institutions), $100.00 per year (US students/residents), $283.00 per year (Canadian individuals), $383.00 per year (Canadian Institutions), $274.00 per year (foreign individuals), $383.00 per year (foreign institutions), and $120.00 per year (international students/residents), $100.00 per year (Canadian students/residents). Foreign air speed delivery is included in all *Clinics'* subscription prices. All prices are subject to change without notice. **POSTMASTER:** Send address changes to *Surgical Pathology Clinics*, Elsevier, 3251 Riverport Lane, Maryland Heights, MO 63043. **Customer Service: 1-800-654-2452 (US). From outside the United States, call 1-314-447-8871. Fax: 1-314-447-8029. E-mail: JournalsCustomerServiceusa@elsevier.com (for print support)** and JournalsOnlineSupport-usa@elsevier.com **(for online support)**.

Reprints. For copies of 100 or more, of articles in this publication, please contact the Commercial Reprints Department, Elsevier Inc., 360 Park Avenue South, New York, NY 10010-1710. Tel. 212-633-3874; Fax: 212-633-3820; E-mail: reprints@elsevier.com.

Surgical Pathology Clinics of North America is covered in *MEDLINE/PubMed (Index Medicus)*.

Contributors

CONSULTING EDITOR

JASON L. HORNICK, MD, PhD
Director of Surgical Pathology and
Immunohistochemistry, Brigham and Women's
Hospital, Professor of Pathology, Harvard
Medical School, Boston, Massachusetts, USA

EDITOR

JUSTIN A. BISHOP, MD
Professor and Chief of Anatomic Pathology,
Jane B. and Edwin P. Jenevein M.D.
Distinguished Chair in Pathology, UT
Southwestern Medical Center, Dallas, Texas

AUTHORS

ABBAS AGAIMY, MD
Institute of Pathology, University Hospital,
Erlangen, Friedrich-Alexander-Universität
Erlangen-Nürnberg (FAU), Erlangen,
Germany

SAMEER ALLAHABADI, BA
Medical Student, Texas Christian University,
University of North Texas Health Science
Center School of Medicine, Fort Worth, Texas,
USA

JUSTIN A. BISHOP, MD
Professor and Chief of Anatomic Pathology,
Jane B. and Edwin P. Jenevein M.D.
Distinguished Chair in Pathology, UT
Southwestern Medical Center, Dallas, Texas

CHRISTOPHER C. GRIFFITH, MD, PhD
The Robert J. Tomsich Pathology and
Laboratory Medicine Institute, Cleveland
Clinic, Cleveland Clinic Head and Neck
Pathology, Cleveland, Ohio, USA

MIN-SHU HSIEH, MD, PhD
Department of Pathology, National Taiwan
University Hospital, Graduate Institute of
Pathology, National Taiwan University College
of Medicine, Taipei, Taiwan

NORA KATABI, MD
Department of Pathology, Memorial Sloan
Kettering Cancer Center, New York, New York,
USA

SAAD A. KHAN, MD
Assistant Professor, Stanford Cancer Institute
and Stanford University, Department of
Medicine-Oncology, Stanford, CA, USA

TOSHITAKA NAGAO, MD, PhD
Professor, Department of Anatomic Pathology,
Tokyo Medical University, Shinjuku-ku, Tokyo,
Japan

MASATO NAKAGURO, MD, PhD
Associate Professor, Department of Pathology
and Laboratory Medicine, Nagoya University
Hospital, Showa-ku, Nagoya, Japan

DOREEN PALSGROVE, MD
Assistant Professor, Department of Pathology,
University of Texas Southwestern Medical
Center, Dallas, Texas, USA

MOBEEN RAHMAN, MD
The Robert J. Tomsich Pathology and
Laboratory Medicine Institute, Cleveland
Clinic, Cleveland Clinic Head and Neck
Pathology, Cleveland, Ohio, USA

ROBERT A. ROBINSON, MD, PhD
Professor, Department of Pathology, University
of Iowa, University of Iowa Carver College of
Medicine, Iowa City, Iowa, USA

LISA M. ROOPER, MD
Assistant Professor, Departments of Pathology
and Oncology, The Johns Hopkins University
School of Medicine, Baltimore, Maryland, USA

LESTER D.R. THOMPSON, MD
Consultant Pathologist, Department of
Pathology, Kaiser Permanente, Woodland
Hills, California, USA

EMILIJA TODOROVIC, MD
Clinical Fellow, Department of Pathology,
University Health Network, Department of
Laboratory Medicine and Pathobiology,
University of Toronto, Toronto, Ontario,
Canada

ILAN WEINREB, MD
Consultant Pathologist, Department of
Pathology, University Health Network,
Department of Laboratory Medicine and
Pathobiology, University of Toronto, Toronto,
Ontario, Canada

RUMEAL D. WHALEY, MD
IU Health Pathology Laboratory, Indiana
University School of Medicine, Indianapolis,
Indiana, USA

BIN XU, MD, PhD
Department of Pathology, Memorial Sloan
Kettering Cancer Center, New York, New York,
USA

JULIA YU FONG CHANG, DDS, MS, PhD
Department of Dentistry, National Taiwan
University Hospital, Department of Dentistry,
Graduate Institute of Clinical Dentistry, School
of Dentistry, National Taiwan University, Taipei,
Taiwan

Contents

Intraductal carcinoma of the salivary gland is a rare tumor characterized by intracystic proliferations of papillary, cribriform, and solid architecture of small uniform epithelial cells, reminiscent of ductal carcinoma in situ of the breast. Recent literature has identified 4 distinctive subtypes: the intercalated duct type, apocrine type, mixed/hybrid type, and oncocytic type, all with corresponding immunohistochemical and molecular findings. Although these tumors are typically in situ, as evidenced by a retained myoepithelial layer, they can demonstrate minimal invasion or, rarely, widespread invasive growth. Their overall prognosis is favorable, with few reported cases of recurrences and nodal metastases but no evidence of distant metastases.

Sclerosing polycystic adenoma (SPA) is the more appropriate name for sclerosing polycystic adenosis. SPA is an uncommon salivary gland lesion with a constellation of unusual histologic findings that were originally interpreted as analogous to breast fibrocystic changes. The histologic findings in SPA include fibrosis, cystic alterations, apocrine metaplasia, and proliferations of ducts, acini, and myoepithelial cells in variable proportions. Because of its unusual mixed histology, SPA may be confused with a variety of lesions, ranging from reactive conditions to benign or even malignant neoplasms. The features of SPA are reviewed, with an emphasis on resolving its differential diagnosis.

Basal cell adenoma (BCA) and basal cell adenocarcinoma (BCAC) are uncommon biphasic salivary gland tumors having morphologic similarities to other biphasic salivary gland neoplasms having differentiation toward the intercalated ducts of the salivary gland. Both tumors show mixtures of trabecular, tubular, solid, and membranous solid patterns. BCAC is separated from BCA primarily by the presence of invasion in the former. The diagnosis of BCA and BCAC is best carried out with hematoxylin and eosin–stained sections and careful attention to detail of tumors in the differential diagnosis, including adenoid cystic carcinoma, pleomorphic adenoma, and epithelial myoepithelial carcinoma.

Sialadenoma papilliferum (SP) is a rare, benign salivary gland neoplasm sharing similar histopathologic features and harboring the same genetic alterations, BRAF V600E or HRAS mutations, with syringocystadenoma papilliferum. SP most commonly occurs in the hard palate and in older adults. Clinically, SP is most likely to be diagnosed as a squamous papilloma. Microscopically, SP shows an exophytic papillary epithelial proliferation and a contiguously endophytic ductal proliferation. Two distinct subtypes are identified: classic SP and oncocytic SP. Conservative surgical treatment seems to be adequate with a low recurrence. SOX10 immunohistochemistry and BRAF analysis may be useful in differential diagnosis.

Papillary lesions of the salivary duct systems are uncommon. They encompass a heterogeneous group of benign, intermediate, and potentially aggressive neoplasms. With a few exceptions, historical descriptive terms such as papillary adenocarcinoma, papillary cystadenocarcinoma, and papillary adenoma are being replaced by defined entities, at same time acknowledging the papillary features as a histologic pattern. The evolving genetic landscape of these lesions increasingly permits their reproducible categorization. This article discusses those papillary proliferations encountered in the salivary glands with a focus on intraductal papillary mucinous neoplasms and cystadenomas. Intraductal carcinomas and sialadenoma papilliferum are addressed in separate articles in this issue.

Myoepithelial carcinoma (MECA) may overlap histologically with other salivary gland neoplasms, especially pleomorphic adenoma. MECA is characterized by cellular, uniform growth of myoepithelial cells and multinodular expansile invasive pattern with zonal cellular distribution. It may arise de novo or in association with pleomorphic adenoma (myoepithelial carcinoma ex pleomorphic adenoma). By immunohistochemistry, MECA is positive for cytokeratins and at least one of the myoepithelial markers, including S100. PLAG1 fusion is the most common genetic alteration. Carcinoma ex pleomorphic adenoma and necrosis correlate with worse clinical outcome in MECA, and necrosis can be used to stratify MECA as high grade.

Lymphoepithelial carcinoma of salivary glands (LECSG) is an uncommon neoplasm. This article summarizes the findings of 438 cases in a review of the literature. Concurrent lymphoepithelial lesions may suggest a primary tumor. The tumor shows a nonkeratinizing carcinoma intimately associated with a rich lymphohistiocytic infiltrate, destroying adjacent salivary gland tissue. Irrespective of race or ethnicity, the tumors usually express Epstein-Barr virus, with Epstein-Barr virus encoded small RNA (EBER) and/or latent membrane protein-1 (LMP-1), although a subset does not. There is an overall good prognosis of about 80% at 5 years.

Epithelial–myoepithelial carcinoma is an uncommon low-grade salivary gland carcinoma. It is classically characterized by biphasic tubular structures composed of inner eosinophilic ductal cells and outer clear myoepithelial cells. In addition, epithelial–myoepithelial carcinoma sometimes shows various histologic features, including a cribriform pattern, basaloid appearance, and sebaceous differentiation. Because clear myoepithelial cells are also noted in other benign and malignant salivary gland tumors, the histologic variety and similarity with other tumor entities make the diagnosis of epithelial–myoepithelial carcinoma challenging. A recent analysis revealed that HRAS hotspot point mutations are specifically identified in epithelial–myoepithelial carcinoma and the assessment of given genes facilitate the correct diagnosis.

Salivary duct carcinoma (SDC) is a rare, aggressive salivary gland malignancy with significant mortality. Morphologically, most tumors are characterized by apocrine differentiation with a typical immunophenotype of androgen receptor positive/gross cystic disease fluid protein positive/estrogen receptor negative/progesterone receptor negative. Several morphologic variants of SDC exist, representing diagnostic pitfalls. Several differential diagnoses should be considered because prognosis, treatment, and management may be different from SDC. For SDC, current treatment strategies are aggressive and commonly include surgical excision with lymph node dissection and adjuvant radiotherapy. Continued research is examining the utility of androgen deprivation therapy and targeted molecular therapy.

Polymorphous adenocarcinoma (PAC) is typically originated from the minor salivary glands and is characterized by cytology uniformity and architectural diversity. PAC commonly harbors PRKD1 E710D mutation. PAC has an excellent prognosis. However, greater than or equal to 10% papillary or greater than or equal to 30% cribriform pattern is an independent adverse prognostic factor. Cribriform adenocarcinoma of salivary gland (CASG) is a controversial entity that is considered within the same histologic spectrum of PAC in current classification schemes; however, it is regarded by some pathologists as a separate entity. CASG shows a propensity to base of tongue location, a lobulated growth pattern, a predominant solid/cribriform architecture, and a high frequency of PRKD1/2/3 fusion.

In recent years, increased molecular testing and improved immunohistochemical panels have facilitated more specific classification of salivary gland carcinomas, leading to recognition of several novel tumor types and unique histologic variants. Sclerosing microcystic adenocarcinoma, microsecretory adenocarcinoma, and secretory myoepithelial carcinoma are three such recently described entities that demonstrate low-grade cytology, production of prominent secretory material, and variable amounts of sclerotic stroma. This review provides a practical overview of these important and overlapping emerging entities in salivary gland pathology with a focus on distinctive histologic features and helpful ancillary studies that differentiate them from a wide range of familiar morphologic mimics.

Salivary gland cancer is a heterogenous group of tumors that presents challenges with both diagnosis and therapy. Recent advances in the classification of salivary gland cancers have led to distinct histologic and genomic criteria that successfully differentiate between cancers with similar clinical behavior and appearance. Genomic abnormalities have led to the emergence of targeted therapies being used in their therapy with drastic improvements in outcomes as well as reductions in treatment-related toxicity. Dramatic results seen with molecular targets, such as HER2, TRK, and others, indicate that this approach has the potential to yield even better treatments for the future.

SURGICAL PATHOLOGY CLINICS

SERIES OF RELATED INTEREST

Clinics in Laboratory Medicine
https://www.labmed.theclinics.com/
Medical Clinics
https://www.medical.theclinics.com/

THE CLINICS ARE AVAILABLE ONLINE!
Access your subscription at:
www.theclinics.com

Preface
Updates on "Under the Radar" Salivary Gland Tumors

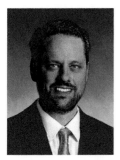

Justin A. Bishop, MD
Editor

There have been a number of exciting advances in salivary gland tumor pathology in the past 10 years. In particular, molecular findings, which have a drastic impact on diagnosis, classification, and even therapy, are advancing at a rapid pace. While considerable attention has been given, appropriately, to relatively common tumors like pleomorphic adenoma, secretory carcinoma, adenoid cystic carcinoma, and mucoepidermoid carcinoma, this issue of *Surgical Pathology Clinics* focuses on the recent discoveries involving salivary gland tumors that are rarer, and therefore, may be less well known.

First, Drs Todorovic and Weinreb examine the enigmatic intraductal carcinoma, a tumor now known to be composed of molecularly distinct entities, which may, in fact, not be intraductal at all. Next, Dr Thompson and I discuss a tumor formerly known as sclerosing polycystic adenosis. Emerging molecular studies have now shown that this lesion is neoplastic and therefore now better known as sclerosing polycystic adenoma. Then, Dr Robinson tackles the topic of basal cell salivary gland tumors, a spectrum of neoplasms that includes basal cell adenoma and basal cell adenocarcinoma, which have overlapping histologic, immunophenotypic, and molecular characteristics. Next, Drs Hsieh, Chang, and I describe sialadenoma papilliferum, a rare oral cavity tumor recently shown to frequently harbor *BRAF* V600E mutations. Dr Agaimy then provides a helpful review of papillary salivary gland neoplasms, a challenging differential diagnosis that includes the newly recognized salivary intraductal papillary mucinous neoplasm. Drs Xu and Katabi delve into myoepithelial carcinoma, a challenging tumor that has emerging genetic findings and many diagnostic pitfalls. Subsequently, Drs Thompson and Whaley provide an updated look at lymphoepithelial carcinoma, a likely underrecognized salivary gland malignancy frequently harboring Epstein-Barr virus. Drs Nakaguro and Nagao then detail the new histologic and molecular findings of epithelial-myoepithelial carcinoma. Following that, Drs Rahman and Griffith deal with one of the most aggressive salivary gland tumors, known as salivary duct carcinoma. Drs Katabi and Xu return with an updated review of polymorphous adenocarcinoma, a salivary gland tumor whose classification remains contentious. Dr Rooper introduces some salivary gland tumors that are so new that they are not yet formally recognized. Finally, Drs Khan and Palsgrove, along with Mr Allahabadi, give us a much-needed oncologist's perspective on salivary gland tumor pathology.

Whether in an academic subspecialized environment where these lesions may be common or in community practice where they are rare, I sincerely hope that the reader finds this review to be useful in her surgical pathology practice.

Justin A. Bishop, MD
UT Southwestern Medical Center
Clements University Hospital UH04.250
6201 Harry Hines Boulevard
Dallas, TX 75390, USA

E-mail address:
Justin.Bishop@utsouthwestern.edu

Surgical Pathology 14 (2021) xi
https://doi.org/10.1016/j.path.2020.12.001
1875-9181/21/© 2020 Published by Elsevier Inc.

surgpath.theclinics.com

Intraductal Carcinomas of the Salivary Gland

Emilija Todorovic, MD[a,b], Ilan Weinreb, MD[a,b,*]

KEYWORDS

• Intraductal carcinoma • NCOA4-RET • Intercalated duct type • TRIM27-RET

Key points

- Intraductal carcinomas of the salivary gland are rare neoplasms with predominantly intraductal growth but also invasive growth.
- They are characterized by intracystic proliferations of papillary, solid, and cribriform architecture as in ductal carcinoma in-situ of the breast.
- The intercalated duct type, apocrine type, mixed type, and oncocytic type now are recognized.
- These tumors are characterized by recurrent RET fusions (*NCOA4-RET* and variants); however, alterations in the *PIK3CA* pathway and *HRAS* mutations are seen in pure apocrine examples associated with salivary duct carcinoma.
- Intraductal carcinoma demonstrates a favorable prognosis.

ABSTRACT

Intraductal carcinoma of the salivary gland is a rare tumor characterized by intracystic proliferations of papillary, cribriform, and solid architecture of small uniform epithelial cells, reminiscent of ductal carcinoma in situ of the breast. Recent literature has identified 4 distinctive subtypes: the intercalated duct type, apocrine type, mixed/hybrid type, and oncocytic type, all with corresponding immunohistochemical and molecular findings. Although these tumors are typically in situ, as evidenced by a retained myoepithelial layer, they can demonstrate minimal invasion or, rarely, widespread invasive growth. Their overall prognosis is favorable, with few reported cases of recurrences and nodal metastases but no evidence of distant metastases.

INTRODUCTION

Intraductal carcinoma of the salivary glands is a rare and enigmatic tumor that bears morphologic resemblance to atypical ductal hyperplasia (ADH) and ductal carcinoma in situ (DCIS) of the breast. The latest World Health Organization (WHO) classification system defines it as a "carcinoma characterized by intracystic/intraductal proliferations of neoplastic epithelial cells."[1] Although the current WHO definition of this tumor is clear and concise, the terminology and characterization of this tumor have not been straightforward. This is evidenced by the fact that intraductal carcinoma has carried many different names since its original description, including low-grade salivary duct carcinoma, low-grade cribriform cystadenocarcinoma, and carcinoma in situ of the salivary gland, among others.[2] Eventually, the term, *intraductal carcinoma*, originally coined by Chen and colleagues,[3] in 1983, when it was first described, has made a comeback in the latest 2017 WHO classification.

Nonetheless, the taxonomy of intraductal carcinomas remains a matter of controversy, as reflected by the frequent terminology changes. Recent literature increasingly recognizes 3 distinct

[a] Department of Laboratory Medicine and Pathobiology, University Health Network, 200 Elizabeth Street, Toronto, Ontario M5G 2C4, Canada; [b] Department of Laboratory Medicine and Pathobiology, University of Toronto, Toronto, Ontario, Canada
* Corresponding author.
E-mail address: ILAN.WEINREB@UHN.CA

Surgical Pathology 14 (2021) 1–15
https://doi.org/10.1016/j.path.2020.09.003
1875-9181/21/© 2021 Elsevier Inc. All rights reserved.

morphologic subtypes of IDC: the intercalated duct type, apocrine type, and hybrid or mixed type (consisting of an admixture of intercalated duct type and apocrine features).[4,5] Additionally, a small series of 5 cases by Nakaguro and colleagues[6] also has proposed the so-called oncocytic variant of intraductal carcinoma due to its prominent oncocytic features. Significantly, the increasing molecular profiling of intraductal carcinomas is demonstrating recurrent molecular alterations, which appear to be specific to each subtype, such as the *NCOA4-RET* rearrangements in the intercalated duct type and *TRIM27-RET* rearrangements predominantly in the mixed subtype.[7] It also is recent that the proposed oncocytic subtype intraductal carcinoma has demonstrated the presence of a *RET* rearrangement with a novel partner (personal communication from Dr Justin Bishop, UT Southwestern Medical Center, 2020). The distinctive morphology and molecular features related to each subtype raise the question if these simply are variants of intraductal carcinoma or if they merit a revised classification as distinctive tumor entities.

The second long-standing controversy related to intraductal carcinomas is their relationship as a precursor lesion to conventional high-grade salivary duct carcinoma. Although most reports in the literature recognize these as distinct tumor entities, recent literature has demonstrated a potential molecular connection between the so-called low-grade apocrine intraductal carcinoma and high-grade conventional salivary duct carcinoma.[4] The fact that many of these cases show microinvasion and rarely show extensive invasion also suggests a potential link to salivary duct carcinoma in some cases.

Herein, the authors discuss the features and controversies related to this rare and unique tumor.

GROSS FEATURES

Intraductal carcinomas occur predominantly in the parotid gland, although they also have been described as arising in the submandibular gland, buccal mucosa, palate, and rarely the lacrimal gland.[3,5,8,9] They also have been reported to arise in intraparotid lymph nodes, hypothetically from salivary ductal inclusions[10] (Fig. 1).

On gross examination, the tumors generally are small and well circumscribed with solid architecture and the formation of variably sized cysts, which can demonstrate hemorrhagic changes. The size may range anywhere between 0.6 cm and 4.6 cm.[2,4,11,12]

MICROSCOPIC FEATURES

At low power, intraductal carcinomas generally are unencapsulated and well circumscribed, with an expansive, multilobular growth (Fig. 2). They are composed of variably sized cysts and ducts with intracystic/intraductal proliferations of small cuboidal cells (Fig. 3). There usually is a variety of architectural patterns seen within the ducts and cysts of each tumor. The typical architectural pattern consists of cribriform structures composed of Roman arc–like bridges (Fig. 4), much like ADH and DCIS of the breast.[7,13] Other architectural patterns also are seen, however: pseudocribriform architecture with slitlike spaces and streaming nuclei (similar to usual ductal hyperplasia of the breast) as well as papillary and anastomosing micropapillary structures with tufting of the surface epithelium (Fig. 5). The vascular cores of the papillae can show prominent hyalinized stroma. Occasionally, the micropapillary tufted forms also can show microvacuolated cells with lipofuscin-like pigment deposition.[7,13] Isolated psammoma bodies may be present.[10] Not

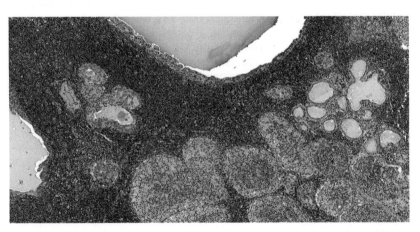

Fig. 1. A case of intraductal carcinoma entirely arising within a lymph node (hematoxylin-eosin, original magnification 4X).

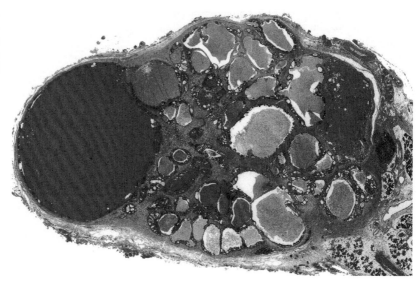

Fig. 2. Intraductal carcinomas are well circumscribed with multilobular growth (hematoxylin-eosin, original magnification 4X).

infrequently, cholesterol clefts, hemorrhage, and dystrophic calcification also can be seen with the tumor. A tumor-associated lymphoid proliferation seen in other salivary gland tumors also has been known to rarely occur, which, when coupled with a papillary architecture, may be a confounding factor in the differential diagnosis with a Warthin tumor.[14] This is an infrequent finding, however, and there are other helpful features to aid in distinguishing between the 2 entities.

The cytomorphologic details of intraductal carcinomas vary predominantly between the intercalated type and apocrine phenotypes. Intercalated ductlike intraductal carcinomas, as the name implies, tend to recapitulate the appearance of normal intercalated ducts. They typically are composed of small cuboidal cells with round to oval nuclei, dispersed chromatin, inconspicuous nucleoli, and eosinophilic to amphophilic

cytoplasm (see **Fig. 3**). Apocrine-type intraductal carcinomas, on the other hand, are characterized by larger cells with ample eosinophilic cytoplasm and round nuclei with prominent nucleoli (**Fig. 6**). Elements of apocrine differentiation, such as decapitation secretions or apocrine snouting, can be seen. Regarding the nuclear grading of intraductal carcinomas, it now is generally accepted that they can have nuclear features that vary from low grade to high grade. Most commonly, intercalated duct–type intraductal carcinoma shows low-grade nuclear features[4]; however, areas with focal cytologic high-grade transformation do occur, especially in cases of invasion.[2,13] Apocrine-type intraductal carcinomas tend to be more frequently high grade, with prominent nuclear pleomorphism, mitotic activity, and comedo-type tumor necrosis similar to the cytomorphologic features of high-grade salivary duct

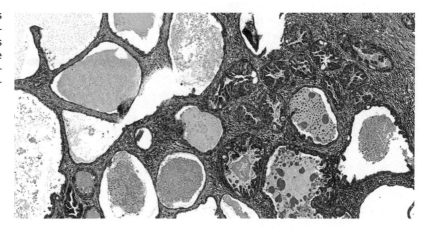

Fig. 3. Cysts and tubules of various sizes with intraluminal proliferations define the appearance of the tumor (hematoxylin-eosin, original magnification 10X).

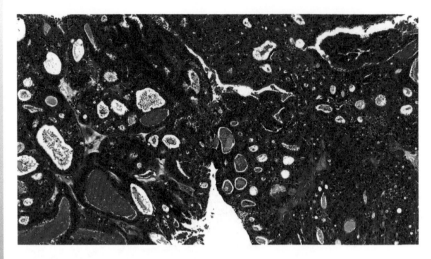

Fig. 4. Solid and cribriform architecture with Roman arch–like bridges reminiscent of ADH/DCIS of the breast can be seen hemotoxylin-eosin, original magnification 10X).

carcinoma, thus explaining the prior reference to these tumors as low-grade salivary duct carcinoma.[15,16] Pure low-grade apocrine-type intraductal carcinomas recently have been described and are extremely rare.[4] Their molecular profile and potential relationship to salivary duct carcinoma are discussed under the heading Molecular Features. Occasionally, intraductal carcinomas with mixed apocrine-intercalated duct–type features can be seen where elements of both subtypes are mixed.[11] The *TRIM27-RET* fusion seems to be correlated to the mixed tumor type.[5,12,17]

Lastly, an oncocytic variant of intraductal carcinoma has been proposed by Nakaguro and colleagues.[6] Their series of 5 cases of intraductal carcinoma were described as composed of cells with "medium-sized round nuclei and abundant granular cytoplasm"[6] (**Fig. 7**). None of the tumors was positive for androgen receptor (AR) or gross cystic disease fluid protein 15 (GCDFP-15) to suggest apocrine morphology. Following the publication of that study and based on an index case, subsequent molecular profiling of 2 of these oncocytic-type cases demonstrated the presence of a novel *RET* rearrangement with an unreported partner to date (personal communication from Dr J. Bishop, University of Texas Southwestern Medical Center) (**Fig. 8**). The novel *RET* fusion associated with the oncocytic variant of intraductal

Fig. 5. Anastomosing micropapillary architecture with a filigree-like pattern can be seen lining the ductal wall (hematoxylin-eosin, original magnification 40X).

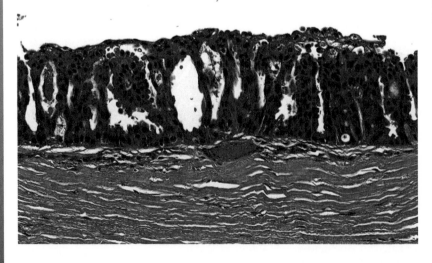

Fig. 6. Apocrine-type intraductal carcinomas show ample eosinophilic cytoplasm, round nuclei with prominent nucleoli and apocrine snouting (hematoxylin-eosin, original magnification 20X).

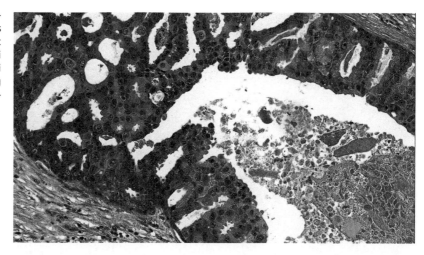

carcinoma may be defining a separate category of intraductal carcinoma. If this were the case, the proposed oncocytic variant certainly would expand the differential diagnosis of intraductal carcinomas to include oncocytic lesions of the salivary gland. Further studies are necessary, however, to definitively categorize and further refine this rare subtype.

As the current terminology implies, intraductal carcinomas are typically in situ tumors, with the intraductal/intracystic tumor cells confined by a myoepithelial cell layer. The myoepithelial layer usually is inconspicuous on hematoxylin-eosin (H&E) examination but becomes apparent on immunohistochemical staining (see heading Immunohistochemistry). Between 20% and 30% of the cases, however, can show microinvasion with an associated background desmoplastic reaction.[5,7,18] This is evidenced by the loss of the myoepithelial layer on immunohistochemistry. Widely invasive growth can occur, although it is less common and has been demonstrated more frequently in the apocrine subtype.[4,5,19] One reported case of a low-grade apocrine-type intraductal carcinoma unusually gave rise to an invasive adenosquamous carcinoma, with subsequent regional lymph node metastasis.[19] Even though it occurs less commonly, intercalated

Fig. 7. Oncocytic-type intraductal carcinoma shows ample granular cytoplasm with a distinctly eosinophilic appearance (hematoxylin-eosin, original magnification 10X). (*Courtesy of* J. Bishop, MD, Dallas, TX.)

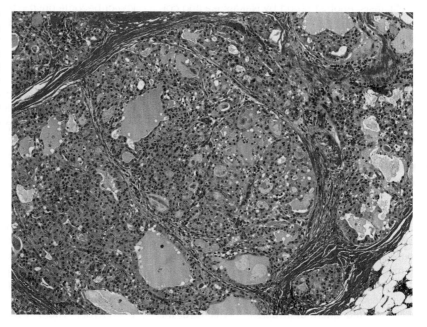

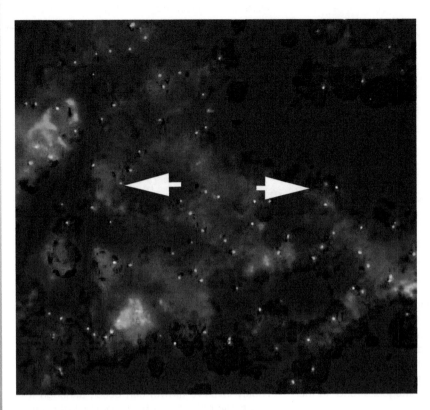

Fig. 8. FISH showing a split signal (*arrows*) for *RET*, indicating a *RET* rearrangement (Fluorescence in-situ hybridization (FISH)). (*Courtesy of* J. Bishop, MD, Dallas, TX.)

duct–type carcinomas also can give rise to an invasive carcinoma with widespread invasion.[5,7,13] One of the cases reported by Skalova and colleagues[5] had an intercalated duct–type carcinoma with widespread invasion and regional lymph node metastasis. Another report by Nakatsuka and colleagues[20] described an intraductal carcinoma with diffuse S100-positive staining giving rise to an infiltrative adenocarcinoma not otherwise specified (NOS). Although the intercalated duct–type characteristic *RET* rearrangements were not known at the time of publication, the immunohistochemical profile and histomorphologic appearance of this tumor were strongly suggestive of an intercalated duct type. The invasive tumor types arising in intercalated duct–type intraductal carcinoma in the literature have been variable. A recent case of an *NCOA4-RET*–positive intercalated duct–type intraductal carcinoma gave rise to an invasive adenocarcinoma, which is a peculiar pattern of invasion. It included a combination of cystic spaces filled with loose micropapillary tuft and detached papillary elements, reminiscent of the spread through air spaces phenomenon seen in lung adenocarcinomas.[7] In contrast, other investigators have described infiltration of solid nests of cells with a limited extent of invasion.[13] Whichever the pattern of invasion, the invasive component may or may not be associated with progression of cytologic features to higher-grade morphology compared with the remainder of the tumor. The same is true for mitotic activity, which may remain low or become brisk in the invasive component.[5,7] Perineural invasion is not a common occurrence in the intraductal carcinomas but has been reported occasionally.

Paradoxically, a point of caution when assessing an intraductal carcinoma is that occasionally a tumor can be distorted and appear invasive but still retain the myoepithelial cell layer (thus remaining in situ). Generally speaking, even with invasive growth, intraductal carcinomas tend to lack other histologic features of aggressive growth, such as a destructive form of invasion or perineural invasion, reflecting their relatively indolent nature. A recent case of a pure intraductal carcinoma known to the authors was found to involve bone (**Fig. 9**). The tumor was originating in the oral cavity minor salivary glands and extensively involved bone. The tumor was well circumscribed with low-grade nuclear features and focal gland distortion. It was diffusely positive for S100 by immunohistochemistry, consistent with an intercalated duct phenotype. There was a focus of squamous

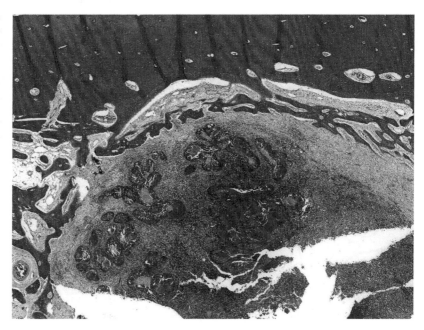

Fig. 9. Well-circumscribed multilobular intraductal carcinoma involving the bone. Despite a myoepithelial layer surrounding the nests, this tumor shows clear bone invasion raising the possibility that all intraductal carcinomas are invasive (hemotoxylin-eosin, original magnification 2X).

metaplastic-like changes, which were suspected to be related to a previous biopsy procedure. The myoepithelial layer was intact even within the bone with focal loss in the metaplastic area. Overall, this phenomenon was unexpected given the low-grade and presumably in situ nature of the lesion.

IMMUNOHISTOCHEMISTRY

Intraductal carcinomas are positive for AE1/AE3, CAM5.2, cytokeratin (CK) 7 (**Fig. 10**), cytokeratin (CK) 19, and epithelial membrane antigen (EMA) in the epithelial cells.[5] The myoepithelial cells are positive for myoepithelial markers, such as p63, calponin, smooth muscle actin (SMA) (**Fig. 11**), CK14, and CK5/6. The p63 immunohistochemical stain typically shows a partially discontinuous myoepithelial cell layer, which should not be interpreted as loss of the layer[5] (**Fig. 12**). A majority of intraductal carcinomas in the literature to date are defined by an intercalated duct phenotype. The epithelial cells are diffusely positive for S100 (**Fig. 13**) and SOX-10 and often positive for mammaglobin.[8] The intercalated duct phenotype is negative for AR and GCDFP-15.

Apocrine intraductal carcinomas, on the other hand, are positive for AR (**Fig. 14**) and GCDFP-15 while S100 negative.[4,11,19] Mixed intercalated duct–type and apocrine tumors can show a combination of AR and GCDFP-15 positivity in the apocrine component and S100 and SOX-10 positivity in the intercalated duct component.[11]

The immunohistochemical profile of the oncocytic variant of intraductal carcinoma from the case series in the literature includes positive staining for AE1/AE3, S100, and mammaglobin and negative staining for AR and GCDFP-15 in the epithelial neoplastic cells.[6] There also was diffusely strong positivity for antimitochondria antibody, supporting the oncocytic changes seen on H&E. The myoepithelial cells stained as expected with myoepithelial markers.

MOLECULAR FEATURES

The molecular landscape of intraductal carcinoma continues to evolve and has garnered considerable attention over the past few years (**Table 1**). As in many salivary gland tumors, recurrent fusions have been detected and the most common are fusions involving the *RET* gene, seen in 23% to 47% of the cases.[7,11,12] The most common is the *NCOA4-RET* fusion (joining exon 7 or 8 of *NCOA4* and exon 12 of *RET* gene), seen in up to 47% of the cases of intraductal carcinoma and typically associated with the intercalated duct type.[5,12] One of the cases with the *NCOA4-RET* fusion (joining exon 6 of *NCOA4* and exon 12 of *RET* gene) demonstrated an intrachromosomal fusion, which could not be detected by fluorescence in situ hybridization (FISH) for *RET* rearrangements; however, it was detected by reverse

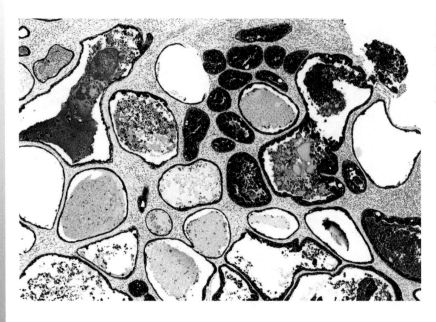

Fig. 10. Immunohistochemical staining for CK7 shows diffuse positivity in the tumor cells (immunohistochemistry, CK7, original magnification 4X).

transcription polymerase chain reaction (RT-PCR). The mixed type of intraductal carcinoma also was shown to harbor this fusion.[7] Mixed intercalated duct/apocrine–type intraductal carcinomas, on the other hand, have shown a *TRIM27-RET* fusion (joining exon 3 of *TRIM27* and exon 12 of *RET* gene) in a subset of cases.[5,11,12] Of the intercalated-type and mixed intraductal carcinomas with the *NCOA4-RET* fusion, approximately 27% have demonstrated invasive growth,

further supporting the notion that these tumors are distinct from salivary duct carcinoma as opposed to representing a precursor lesion.[5,7,12] Two rare fusions, *TUT1-ETV5* and *KIAA1217-RET*, also have been reported by Skalova and colleagues[5] in intraductal carcinoma with invasive growth; however, these have not been demonstrated in other salivary gland cancers to date. The *KIAA1217-RET* fusion, however, previously was reported in lung adenocarcinoma, where it

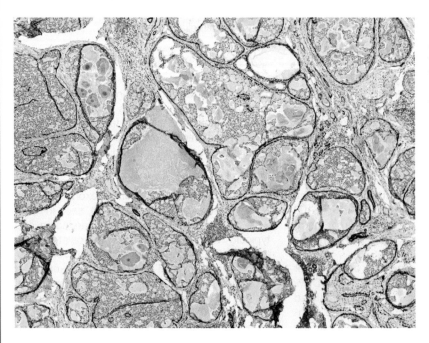

Fig. 11. Immunohistochemical staining for SMA shows an intact myoepithelial layer (immunohistochemistry, SMA, original magnification 4X).

Fig. 12. Immunohistochemical staining for p63 shows a discontinuous rim of myoepithelial cells throughout (immunohistochemistry, p63, original magnification 10X).

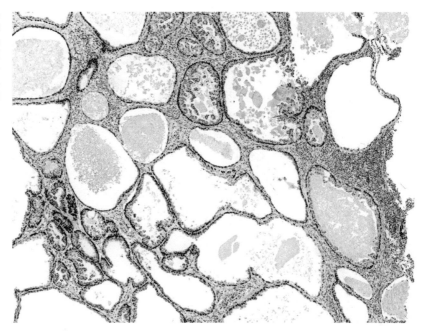

was suggested to represent a novel oncogenic driver gene conferring sensitivity to targeted lung therapy.[21] The significance of this in salivary gland carcinoma is unknown at this time.

In contrast, apocrine-type IDCs, whether with high-grade or low-grade nuclear features, tend not to harbor fusions but rather show a molecular profile similar to salivary duct carcinoma. They were shown to have *PIK3CA* and *HRAS* (p.Gly13Arg) mutations and *TP53* loss.[4] Other findings included mutations in *ATM* and *SPEN*. This particular molecular profile further raises the question whether apocrine intraductal carcinomas are in fact precursor lesions to conventional salivary duct carcinoma. The literature is divided in this regard, however, with a tendency

Fig. 13. Intercalated duct type showing diffuse S100 positivity (immunohistochemistry, S100, original magnification 4X).

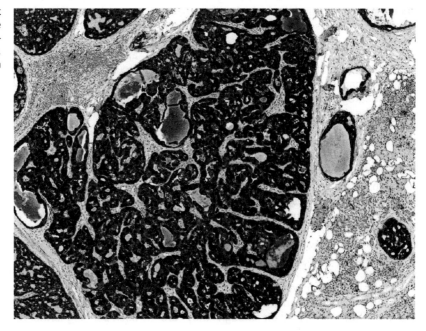

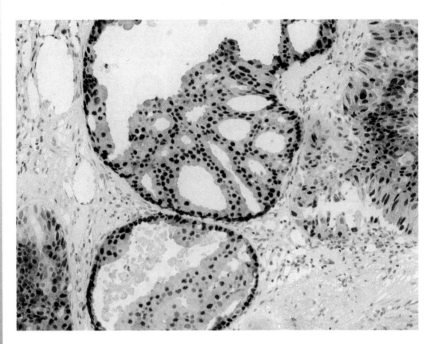

Fig. 14. Apocrine type showing diffuse AR positivity (immunohistochemistry, androgen receptor, original magnification 20X).

toward the 2 being separate entities. Weinreb and colleagues[7] demonstrated the presence of recurrent hotspot mutations in *HRAS* and *PIK3CA* in 2 cases of salivary duct carcinoma with a low-grade intraductal component. Both cases also demonstrated, however, the presence of 2 nonrecurring fusions *DFFA-ARID1A* and *KIF13B-EPB41L4B*, respectively. The case of the *KIF13B-EPB41L4B* fusion showed a predominant low-grade to intermediate-grade intraductal component, not typical of salivary duct carcinoma. Because these cases also demonstrated concurrent alteration in *HRAS* and *PIK3CA*, however, which otherwise were found in cases of other features of conventional salivary duct carcinoma, the belief was that these are best categorized as salivary duct carcinoma, despite the low-grade intraductal component. The notion that intraductal carcinoma and salivary duct carcinoma are separate entities also is supported by a recent study by Skalova and colleagues.[5] They detected an *NCOA4-RET* fusion in widely invasive intraductal carcinomas whereas none of the salivary duct carcinomas was positive for this fusion. In that publication, the investigators proposed reclassifying intraductal carcinomas with this phenotype as noninvasive versus invasive intercalated duct carcinoma.[5] The occurrence of pure intraductal carcinomas in lymph nodes and invading bone, however, also led to the notion that these lesions are not truly in situ even though they are intraductal. This also is supported by the fact that most cases form a mass rather than following the preexisting ductal system the way a diffuse DCIS in the breast does. Further characterization of more cases is necessary to determine whether all intraductal carcinomas should be considered invasive and whether the myoepithelial layer, therefore, is neoplastic, or alternatively whether they represent non-neoplastic myoepithelial cells of preexisting ducts, as has been the traditional thinking.

Bishop and colleagues recently published a small case series of 3 cases of pure low-grade apocrine intraductal carcinoma that share a molecular profile and immunophenotype with salivary duct carcinoma (see **Table 1**).[4]This brought about the possibility that low-grade apocrine intraductal carcinomas are closely related to salivary duct carcinoma. This did not change the prevailing stance in the literature, however, that intraductal carcinomas and high-grade salivary duct carcinoma merit distinct diagnostic categories due to their different clinicopathologic features and biologic potential.

For the time being, further studies are needed. What is increasingly apparent, however, is that intraductal carcinomas likely have several distinct subtypes: the intercalated duct type, apocrine type, mixed type, and oncocytic type. Whether these will merit a separate classification within future WHO classification systems remains to be seen pending further research.

Table 1 Intraductal carcinoma subtype classification comparison				
	Intercalated Duct Type	**Apocrine Type**	**Mixed Type**	**Oncocytic Type**[a]
Histomorphology— low power	Well-circumscribed, multilobulated, basophilic to amphophilic	Well-circumscribed, multilobulated, eosinophilic	Well-circumscribed, multilobulated, combined elements of intercalated duct type and apocrine type	Well-circumscribed, multilobulated, eosinophilic
Histomorphology— high power	Small cuboidal cells with round to oval nuclei, discrete nucleoli and eosinophilic to amphophilic cytoplasm Typically low-grade	Intermediate to large cells with round nuclei, open chromatin, prominent nucleoli and ample eosinophilic granular cytoplasm Decapitation secretions can be seen High-grade forms more frequent Pure low-grade forms can be seen	Elements of both the intercalated duct and apocrine types admixed together	Intermediate cells with medium-sized round nuclei and abundant granular cytoplasm
Immuno histochemical findings	S100, SOX-10 + Mammaglobin + GCDFP15 – AR –	S100, SOX-10 – GCDFP15- + AR +	S100, SOX + GCDFP-15 + AR +	S100, SOX10 + GCDFP-15 – AR –
Myoepithelial markers: p63 + (discontinuous) CK14 Calponin CK5/6 SMA All markers are intact in pure intraductal carcinomas across subtypes and lost in invasive foci			All markers can be patchy or diffusely positive.	
Molecular alterations	*NCOA4-RET* fusion 42.2%–47%[5,7,12] *TUT1-ETV6*[5] *KIAA1217-RET*[5]	*HRAS* *PIK3CA* *PTEN* *SPEN* *ATM* *TP53 copy number loss*	*TRIM27-RET* fusion *NCOA4-RET*	*X-RET*[b]

[a] This subtype is rare in literature, with 5 reported cases to date and 2 additional cases known to the authors.
[b] The fusion partner in this novel subtype currently has not been reported in the literature.

DIFFERENTIAL DIAGNOSIS

The differential diagnosis of intraductal carcinoma includes benign and malignant entities. The benign entities include cystadenoma and sclerosing polycystic adenoma whereas the malignant diagnoses include cystadenocarcinoma, salivary duct carcinoma, acinic cell carcinoma with papillary morphology, and secretory carcinoma.

Cystadenomas of the salivary gland are rare benign salivary gland neoplasms characterized by a unicystic or multicystic growth pattern where the cyst walls are lined by intraluminal papillary proliferations.[1] The lining epithelium is predominantly oncocytic by differentiation; however, epidermoid, mucinous, and apocrine changes can be seen in varying proportions.[22] There is no evidence of cytologic atypia, mitotic activity, or invasive growth that can be seen in intraductal carcinomas nor is there typically evidence of diffuse S100 positivity as would be expected in an intercalated duct–type intraductal carcinoma.[18] Their appearance can be similar to a Warthin tumor albeit without the characteristic lymphoid stroma. There is tremendous variability in cystadenoma morphology and interobserver variability, however, in the ways they are diagnosed. It could be argued that it might be challenging to differentiate cystadenomas from the proposed oncocytic variant of intraductal carcinoma; however, complex internal architecture resembling ADH, which typically is seen in intraductal carcinomas, is a rare occurrence in cystadenomas.[6,23] Furthermore, cystadenomas showing morphology reminiscent of ADH tend to be negative for S100 and GCDFP-15, thus allowing differentiation between the 2 entities.

Sclerosing polycystic adenoma (formerly known as sclerosing polycystic adenosis) is another benign neoplastic lesion that might be challenging to distinguish from intraductal carcinoma. These lesions are well-circumscribed lobular admixtures of cystic ducts and serous acini with prominent hypereosinophilic granules.[1] Features of apocrine differentiation are a common occurrence and the intraluminal epithelial proliferation might be prominent, drawing resemblance to low-grade ductal carcinoma of the breast and thus intraductal carcinoma of salivary gland as well. To further add to the confusion, these show an intact myoepithelial layer. Recent literature has described the occurrence of genetic alterations in the *PIK3CA* pathway, similar to a subset of the apocrine subtype of intraductal carcinoma and salivary duct carcinoma.[24] This raises the question of whether sclerosing polycystic adenoma is in fact on the spectrum with the apocrine-type intraductal carcinoma. Until this is definitively determined, the presence of an invasive component and absence of hypereosinophilic granules in acini would favor an intraductal carcinoma. Both tumor types have been described with high-grade carcinoma in situ.[25]

Salivary duct carcinoma is a highly aggressive and common malignant tumor of the salivary gland, defined by its apocrine morphology and supported by consistent positive staining for AR and GCDFP-15.[1] Due to its aggressive nature, it is an important differential diagnosis for apocrine intraductal carcinoma with which it shares the apocrine features and the immunohistochemical staining pattern. Given the similarities, it is not surprising that intraductal carcinomas previously were referred to as low-grade salivary duct carcinoma.[2,13,18,19] Unlike salivary duct carcinoma, however, which shows widespread infiltrative growth, apocrine intraductal carcinomas generally are well circumscribed with a multilobular growth pattern and lack of invasive growth (if purely in situ). Even if invasive growth is present, the invasive foci typically tend to remain focal and contained (see previous heading Microscopic Features). Moreover, perineural invasion is a rare occurrence, a feature that frequently is seen in salivary duct carcinoma. Relying on cytomorphologic features for the distinction between these 2 entities may or may not be helpful. It now generally is accepted that the cytomorphology of intraductal carcinoma can range from low grade to high grade, with high-grade cases demonstrating prominent nuclear pleomorphism, mitotic figures, and comedo-type tumor necrosis.[1,16] The instances of pure high-grade salivary duct carcinoma in situ without any invasion are rare but have been reported previously by Simpson and colleagues,[15] where the tumors were positive for CK7, AR, and GCDFP-15. Moreover, they retained a myoepithelial cell layer demonstrated by immunohistochemistry throughout, all of which are features consistent with what is now known to be the apocrine-type of intraductal carcinoma. One of the patients in that article had a reported 8-year follow-up free of disease recurrence.[15]

Either way, this differential diagnosis reiterates the importance of entirely submitting and examining entirely an apocrine intraductal lesion to rule out features of aggressive growth, which might suggest that a salivary duct carcinoma. Conventional salivary duct carcinoma with an adjacent intraductal component of growth is not an uncommon occurrence, and prior studies have sought to examine this relationship and how to best categorize these lesions. Furthermore, as described under the previous heading Molecular Features, apocrine intraductal carcinomas and salivary duct carcinomas have been found to share alterations in the *PIK3CA* and *PTEN* genes.[4] Several investigators have agreed that these cases still be categorized as conventional salivary duct carcinoma for now, in line with their aggressive histomorphologic features and biologic potential.[4,5,7,25,26] This reinforces the point that intraductal carcinomas, regardless of subtype or presence of invasive growth, still are relatively indolent malignancies, irrespective of their molecular similarities to salivary duct carcinoma. Thus, they ought to be treated as distinct entities.

Cystadenocarcinoma of the salivary gland is a rare and nebulous tumor category, with a cystic and predominantly papillary architecture reminiscent of intraductal carcinoma, which is why intraductal carcinomas previously were referred to as low-grade cribriform cystadenocarcinoma. These tumors typically have a low-grade appearance and tend to consist of small cuboidal cells with round nuclei and rare mitotic activity. In contrast to intraductal carcinomas, however, they demonstrate prominent infiltrative growth and, importantly, a lack of a myoepithelial cell layer.[27] This can be demonstrated easily 'by performing immunohistochemical staining for myoepithelial cell markers.

Acinic cell carcinoma, particularly one with a papillary cystic architecture, may resemble an intercalated duct–type intraductal carcinoma. Acinic cell carcinomas, however, are negative for staining with S100, which is typically positive in the intraductal carcinoma.

Secretory carcinoma is an important differential diagnosis because occasional intercalated-type intraductal carcinomas can show cystic architecture with papillary growth and vacuolated cytoplasm in the tumor cells. Coupled with S100 positivity in both tumor types, this can be a challenging differential diagnosis. None of the intercalated intraductal carcinomas, however, demonstrates the recurrent t(12;15) (p13;q25), translocation resulting in the *ETV6-NTRK3* fusion, which characterizes secretory carcinoma.[12,27] Rare secretory carcinomas have demonstrated *ETV6-RET* fusions,[28] a finding not described in intraductal carcinomas despite the shared *RET* rearrangement.

PROGNOSIS

Intraductal carcinomas are characterized by relatively indolent behavior and a generally favorable prognosis. To date, no intraductal carcinomas, irrespective of grade without invasive growth, have demonstrated definitive recurrence or distant metastases.[2,7,13,18,25] A small number of cases in the published literature to date have demonstrate invasive growth, with several reported cases of intercalated duct–type intraductal carcinoma showing widespread invasion.[5,18,19] One of these cases, confirmed to have the *NCOA4-RET* fusion, also demonstrated regional lymph node metastases. Outcome data are not available for this patient. Another reported case of an invasive adenosquamous carcinoma arising from an intraductal carcinoma with apocrine features also showed a single nodal metastasis, but this patient was free of disease at 91 months' follow-up.[19] The follow-up time of cases reported in the literature has ranged between 3 months and 19 years.[18] A single publication described 3 cases of high-grade intraductal salivary gland carcinoma, where 1 patient had a recurrence after a partial parotidectomy whereas another patient had a recurrence following transformation of an intraductal to invasive carcinoma.[29] However, it is unclear whether the tumours in that study represented an intraductal carcinoma, salivary duct carcinoma or adenocarcinoma NOS. Either way, in both instances, the tumors were incompletely removed on initial surgery and this may explain the recurrence. Long-term follow-up was not available for longer than 3 months for 1 of the patients.

Overall, the prognosis of these tumors is favorable; however, further studies and longer follow-up are necessary to characterize their long-term prognosis. Currently, conservative excision with clear margins appears to be adequate treatment, although prior treatment modalities have included radiotherapy and chemotherapy (employed in the case of invasive adenosquamous carcinoma).[18] In terms of future directions, the frequent presence of *RET* rearrangements renders it a possibility that these tumors may respond to *RET* inhibitor therapy as is seen in a subset of lung adenocarcinomas.[5] Further studies are needed, however, to determine the potential therapeutic benefit and which patients would get treated, given the generally indolent nature of this tumor category.

SUMMARY

Intraductal carcinomas are rare and peculiar salivary gland tumors with a dominant intraductal growth component and relatively indolent behavior. Along with the characteristic morphology and immunohistochemical profile, recent molecular characterization has demonstrated recurrent *RET* rearrangements, which are defining several different subtypes of intraductal carcinoma. Although these tumors are believed to be distinct from salivary duct carcinoma, recent developments have shown that they demonstrate similar molecular features in a subset of cases. Nonetheless, recognition of these interesting tumors among several differential diagnoses remains important given their favorable prognosis. Further molecular characterization and more case series of intraductal carcinoma might continue to shed more light on these enigmatic entities.

CLINICS CARE POINTS

- Intraductal carcinomas are rare tumors that are effectively in situ carcinomas with an excellent prognosis.

- No true, purely intraductal carcinomas (absent invasion) have demonstrated a recurrence or metastatic potential to date.

- Complete surgical excision of pure intraductal lesions should be considered sufficient therapy at this time, with the caveat that the lesion must be submitted entirely for histologic examination in order to definitively rule out invasion.

- The frequent presence of *RET* rearrangements in intraductal carcinomas may suggest a potential role for *RET* inhibitor therapy; however, further studies are needed.

DISCLOSURE

The authors have nothing to disclose.

REFERENCES

1. El-Naggar A. WHO classification of head and neck tumours. 4th edition. Lyon (France): International Agency for Research on Cancer (IARC); 2017.
2. Delgado R, Klimstra D, Albores-Saavedra J. Low grade salivary duct carcinoma. A distinctive variant with a low grade histology and a predominant intraductal growth pattern. Cancer 1996;78(5):958–67.
3. Chen KT. Intraductal carcinoma of the minor salivary gland. J Laryngol Otol 1983;97(2):189–91.
4. Bishop JA, Gagan J, Krane JF, et al. Low-grade Apocrine Intraductal Carcinoma: Expanding the Morphologic and Molecular Spectrum of an Enigmatic Salivary Gland Tumor. Head Neck Pathol 2020. https://doi.org/10.1007/s12105-020-01128-0, [Online ahead of print].
5. Skalova A, Ptakova N, Santana T, et al. NCOA4-RET and TRIM27-RET Are Characteristic Gene Fusions in Salivary Intraductal Carcinoma, Including Invasive and Metastatic Tumors: Is "Intraductal" Correct? Am J Surg Pathol 2019;43(10):1303–13.
6. Nakaguro M, Urano M, Suzuki H, et al. Low-grade intraductal carcinoma of the salivary gland with prominent oncocytic change: a newly described variant. Histopathology 2018;73(2):314–20.
7. Weinreb I, Bishop JA, Chiosea SI, et al. Recurrent RET Gene Rearrangements in Intraductal Carcinomas of Salivary Gland. Am J Surg Pathol 2018;42(4):442–52.
8. Nojima J, Nakahira M, Yamaguchi H, et al. An extremely rare salivary gland tumor: intraductal carcinoma of the buccal mucosa. Int Cancer Conf J 2016;5(1):53–6.
9. Bursztyn LL, Hyrcza MD, Allen LH, et al. Low-grade intraductal carcinoma of the lacrimal gland. Orbit 2014;33(2):135–8.
10. Weinreb I. Intraductal carcinoma of salivary gland (so-called low-grade cribriform cystadenocarcinoma) arising in an intraparotid lymph node. Head Neck Pathol 2011;5(3):321–5.
11. Lu H, Graham RP, Seethala R, et al. Intraductal Carcinoma of Salivary Glands Harboring TRIM27-RET Fusion with Mixed Low Grade and Apocrine Types. Head Neck Pathol 2020;14(1):239–45.
12. Skalova A, Vanecek T, Uro-Coste E, et al. Molecular Profiling of Salivary Gland Intraductal Carcinoma Revealed a Subset of Tumors Harboring NCOA4-RET and Novel TRIM27-RET Fusions: A Report of 17 cases. Am J Surg Pathol 2018;42(11):1445–55.
13. Brandwein-Gensler M, Hille J, Wang BY, et al. Low-grade salivary duct carcinoma: description of 16 cases. Am J Surg Pathol 2004;28(8):1040–4.
14. Nishijima T, Yamamoto H, Nakano T, et al. Low-grade intraductal carcinoma (low-grade cribriform cystadenocarcinoma) with tumor-associated lymphoid proliferation of parotid gland. Pathol Res Pract 2017;213(6):706–9.
15. Simpson RH, Desai S, Di Palma S. Salivary duct carcinoma in situ of the parotid gland. Histopathology 2008;53(4):416–25.
16. Cheuk W, Miliauskas JR, Chan JK. Intraductal carcinoma of the oral cavity: a case report and a reappraisal of the concept of pure ductal carcinoma in situ in salivary duct carcinoma. Am J Surg Pathol 2004;28(2):266–70.
17. Dwojak S, Bhattacharyya N. Racial disparities in preventable risk factors for head and neck cancer. Laryngoscope 2017;127(5):1068–72.
18. Kuo YJ, Weinreb I, Perez-Ordonez B. Low-grade salivary duct carcinoma or low-grade intraductal carcinoma? Review of the literature. Head Neck Pathol 2013;7(Suppl 1):S59–67.
19. Weinreb I, Tabanda-Lichauco R, Van der Kwast T, et al. Low-grade intraductal carcinoma of salivary gland: report of 3 cases with marked apocrine differentiation. Am J Surg Pathol 2006;30(8):1014–21.

20. Nakatsuka S, Harada H, Fujiyama H, et al. An invasive adenocarcinoma of the accessory parotid gland: a rare example developing from a low-grade cribriform cystadenocarcinoma? Diagn Pathol 2011;6:122.

21. Lee MS, Kim RN, Hoseok I, et al. Identification of a novel partner gene, KIAA1217, fused to RET: Functional characterization and inhibitor sensitivity of two isoforms in lung adenocarcinoma. Oncotarget 2016;7(24):36101–14.

22. Tjioe KC, de Lima HG, Thompson LD, et al. Papillary Cystadenoma of Minor Salivary Glands: Report of 11 Cases and Review of the English Literature. Head Neck Pathol 2015;9(3):354–9.

23. Fahim L, Weinreb I, Alexander C, et al. Epithelial proliferation in small ducts of salivary cystadenoma resembling atypical ductal hyperplasia of breast. Head Neck Pathol 2008;2(3):213–7.

24. Bishop JA, Gagan J, Baumhoer D, et al. Sclerosing Polycystic "Adenosis" of Salivary Glands: A Neoplasm Characterized by PI3K Pathway Alterations More Correctly Named Sclerosing Polycystic Adenoma. Head Neck Pathol 2019;14(3):630–6.

25. Laco J, Podhola M, Dolezalova H. Low-grade cribriform cystadenocarcinoma of the parotid gland: a neoplasm with favorable prognosis, distinct from salivary duct carcinoma. Int J Surg Pathol 2010; 18(5):369–73.

26. Bahrami A, Perez-Ordonez B, Dalton JD, et al. An analysis of PLAG1 and HMGA2 rearrangements in salivary duct carcinoma and examination of the role of precursor lesions. Histopathology 2013; 63(2):250–62.

27. Skalova A, Vanecek T, Sima R, et al. Mammary analogue secretory carcinoma of salivary glands, containing the ETV6-NTRK3 fusion gene: a hitherto undescribed salivary gland tumor entity. Am J Surg Pathol 2010;34(5):599–608.

28. Skalova, et al. Molecular Profiling of Mammary Analog Secretory Carcinoma Revealed a Subset of Tumors Harboring a Novel ETV6-RET translocation: Report of 10 cases. Am J Surg Pathol 2018;42(2): 234–46.

29. Anderson, et al. Intraductal carcinoma of major salivary gland. Cancer 1992;69(3):609–14.

Sclerosing Polycystic Adenoma

Justin A. Bishop, MD[a],*, Lester D.R. Thompson, MD[b]

KEYWORDS

- Sclerosing polycystic adenoma • Sclerosing polycystic adenosis • Salivary glands • Parotid gland
- PI3 kinase

Key points

- Sclerosing polycystic adenoma (SPA), formerly sclerosing polycystic adenosis, was originally believed to be analogous to breast fibrocystic changes.
- SPA is characterized by varying degrees of sclerosis, cystic changes, and proliferations of various salivary gland epithelial elements.
- SPA frequently exhibits apocrine intraductal proliferations resembling breast ductal carcinoma in situ.
- SPA is a neoplastic process harboring genetic alterations in the PI3 kinase pathway, similar to salivary duct carcinoma.
- SPA is benign, occasionally recurring locally. Cases of carcinoma arising in SPA are rare.

ABSTRACT

Sclerosing polycystic adenoma (SPA) is the more appropriate name for sclerosing polycystic adenosis. SPA is an uncommon salivary gland lesion with a constellation of unusual histologic findings that were originally interpreted as analogous to breast fibrocystic changes. The histologic findings in SPA include fibrosis, cystic alterations, apocrine metaplasia, and proliferations of ducts, acini, and myoepithelial cells in variable proportions. Because of its unusual mixed histology, SPA may be confused with a variety of lesions, ranging from reactive conditions to benign or even malignant neoplasms. The features of SPA are reviewed, with an emphasis on resolving its differential diagnosis.

INTRODUCTION

Sclerosing polycystic adenoma (SPA) is a salivary gland neoplasm first described as a distinct entity in 1996 as sclerosing polycystic adenosis, originally thought to be analogous to breast fibrocystic changes.[1,2] The concept of SPA being a nonneoplastic lesion persisted along with the adenosis terminology for more than 2 decades, and was included in the most recent World Health Organization (WHO) classification of salivary gland tumors.[2] However, there is now considerable evidence to suggest that SPA is a neoplasm, and is best regarded as an adenoma.[3,4]

SPA is rare, with fewer than 100 reported cases in the literature.[1,2,4–11] Most SPAs (around 70%) arise in the parotid gland, with occasional cases seen in the submandibular glands or oral cavity.[1,2,5–8,11,12] Rare SPAs have been reported to arise in the sinonasal tract or lacrimal glands.[9,13,14] SPA typically presents in patients as a painless, slow-growing mass. It develops over a wide age range (7–84 years), with a mean age of approximately 40 years at initial presentation.[1,2,5–12] SPA arises slightly more frequently in women than in men (1.3:1).[1,2,5–11]

a Department of Pathology, UT Southwestern Medical Center, 6201 Harry Hines Boulevard, Dallas, TX 75390, USA; b Department of Pathology, Kaiser Permanente, 5601 De Soto Avenue, Woodland Hills, CA 91365, USA
* Corresponding author.
E-mail address: justin.bishop@utsouthwestern.edu

Surgical Pathology 14 (2021) 17–24
https://doi.org/10.1016/j.path.2020.09.004

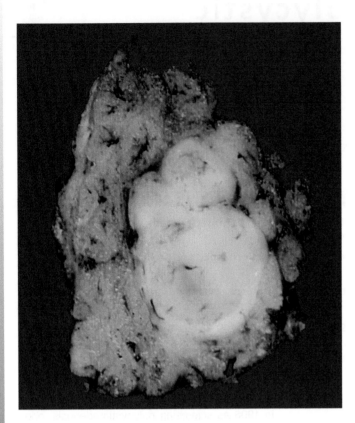

Fig. 1. The macroscopic appearance of SPA is nonspecific, usually consisting of a well-circumscribed tan-white nodule within the otherwise unremarkable parotid parenchyma.

GROSS FEATURES

Grossly, SPA is nonspecific. It consists of a well-circumscribed, firm, tan-white nodule ranging from 1 to 12 cm (**Fig. 1**). Lesions often have a multicystic gross cut surface.

MICROSCOPIC FEATURES

At low power, SPA usually appears well circumscribed and is often encapsulated (**Fig. 2**), frequently containing cystically dilated ducts (see **Fig. 2**A). Some cases have prominent fatty stromal metaplasia; when this feature is present, it may falsely give the impression of an infiltrative process (**Fig. 3**A). Most SPAs have bands of hyalinized fibrosis compartmentalizing the tumor into vague lobules (see **Fig. 2**B).

At medium and high power, SPA is characterized by its mixture of cell types. SPA contains various proliferations of ducts, myoepithelial cells, and acini. The ducts range from small ductules to large cystic spaces. The ductal cells often show apocrine or xanthomatous cytoplasmic alterations (**Fig. 4**). The tumor cysts frequently contain luminal secretions and/or foamy macrophages. The lesional myoepithelial cells are usually subtle, found surrounding the ductal spaces (**Fig. 5**A), but are occasionally more prominent (**Fig. 5**B). The lesional acini may appear normal, but are often filled with large, hypereosinophilic granules or hyaline globules (**Fig. 6**). These globules may represent altered zymogen granules. The acini of SPA often blend with small ductules (see **Fig. 5**A).

Most SPAs show intraductal neoplasia that is usually apocrine and, by itself, indistinguishable from apocrine forms of intraductal carcinoma. Usually the apocrine neoplasia is low grade, resembling breast atypical ductal hyperplasia or low-grade ductal carcinoma in situ with monotonous cells arranged in rigid bridges (**Fig. 7**A). However, the intraductal tumor is occasionally high grade with increased mitoses and comedo-type necrosis, resembling salivary duct carcinoma (**Fig. 7**B). Although they can be atypical or even frankly malignant, these ductal proliferations are almost always completely confined to the ductal system. Only 1 case of invasive carcinoma has been reported to have arisen from SPA.[10] Areas of intralesional sclerosis are common, and should not be misinterpreted as invasive carcinoma (**Fig. 8**).[15]

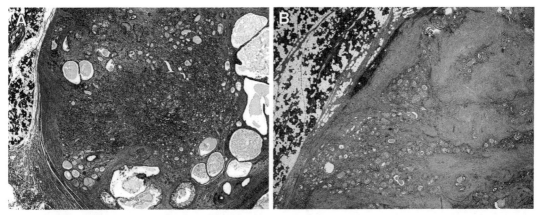

Fig. 2. (*A, B*) The typical low-power appearance of SPA is that of an encapsulated, well-circumscribed tumor with varying degrees of hyalinizing fibrosis and cystic spaces.

It must be emphasized that the histologic appearance of SPA is variable. There are cases that lack 1 or more of the classic features (eg, paucicystic SPA [see **Fig. 3**B], or SPA lacking fibrosis or apocrine changes).[15] The most helpful histologic features are the hypereosinophilic granules and the mixture of different cell types.

PATHOLOGIC KEY FEATURES

The key pathologic features are listed in **Box 1**.

ANCILLARY STUDIES

IMMUNOHISTOCHEMISTRY

Each cellular component (ductal cells, acinar cells, myoepithelial cells) of SPA generally shows its expected immunophenotype (**Fig. 9**). SOX10 highlights small ductules, myoepithelial cells, and acini. Interestingly, the acinar cell marker DOG1 is often weak and focal in the altered acini of SPA. Myoepithelial cell markers such as SMA, p40, calponin, and S100 protein are helpful to highlight the intact myoepithelial cell layer surrounding each duct and the apocrine ductal proliferations. As expected, the apocrine ductal tumor cells are positive for androgen receptor and GCDFP-15.

MOLECULAR TESTING

One study, by Skalova and colleagues,[6] reported X-chromosome inactivation in all tested cases using polymorphism of the human androgen receptor, suggesting that SPA is a neoplastic process. Because intraductal lesions are so common in SPA, this study left it unresolved as to whether the entire lesion was neoplastic or just the ductal proliferations.

More recently, Bishop and colleagues analyzed SPAs with next-generation sequencing and found that all, even those that lacked any intraductal

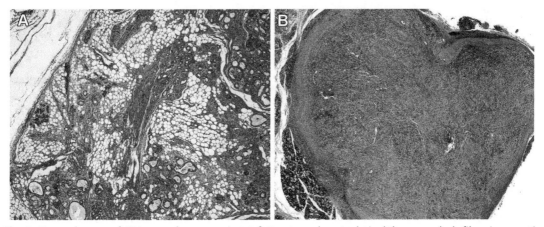

Fig. 3. Unusual cases of SPA may show prominent fatty stromal metaplasia (*A*) or may lack fibrosis or cystic changes (*B*).

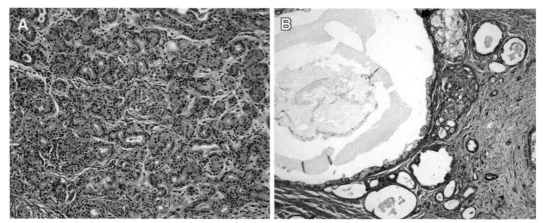

Fig. 4. The ducts of SPA range from small tubules resembling intercalated ducts (*A*) to variably sized cysts often lined by apocrine or xanthomatous cells (*B*).

proliferations, harbored mutations in the phosphatidylinositol 3 (PI3) kinase pathway, most frequently *PTEN*.[4] This finding is strong evidence that SPA is a neoplasm with genetics similar to apocrine intraductal carcinoma or salivary duct carcinoma. Interestingly, PTEN immunohistochemistry showed loss of expression in all ductal and acinar cell types, but expression was retained in the lesional myoepithelial cells. This finding suggests that the myoepithelial cells of SPA may be nonneoplastic, further tying SPA to apocrine intraductal carcinoma as possibly related entities.

DIFFERENTIAL DIAGNOSIS

SPA is confounding to pathologists unfamiliar with this rare tumor type because it shares features with nonneoplastic processes in benign or even malignant salivary gland neoplasms. Accordingly, its differential diagnosis is often broad.

The ductal dilatation and fibrosis seen in SPA frequently suggest polycystic/dysgenetic disease or nonspecific sialofibrosis with salivary duct cysts. In contrast with those processes, SPA is well circumscribed and does not involve the entire gland. Moreover, SPA is usually clearly proliferative. Further, polycystic/dysgenetic disease is usually bilateral and seen at a much younger age than most cases of SPA.[16]

In SPAs with a prominent lipomatous stroma, sialolipoma (a lipoma with entrapped salivary ducts, acini, and myoepithelial cells) is a consideration. However, in sialolipoma, the epithelial elements are either normal or atrophic in appearance, very different from the proliferative nature of SPA.[17]

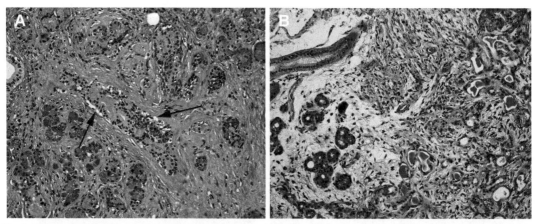

Fig. 5. The myoepithelial cells in SPA are situated around the ductal component and are typically subtle and indistinct (*arrows*). Note how the small ductules blend into lesional acini (*A*). On occasion, the myoepithelial cells (in this case, spindled cells in a myxoid background) can be focally prominent (*B*). The presence of abnormal acini (*left*) help distinguish this from pleomorphic adenoma.

Fig. 6. Acinar cells are a classic histologic feature of SPA. Although some have a typical appearance with fine, basophilic granules (*left*), many of the granules are large and brightly eosinophilic (*right*).

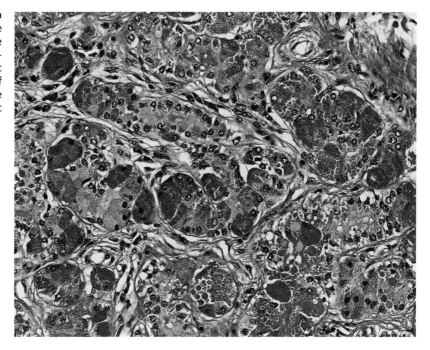

SPA shows overlapping histologic features with pleomorphic adenoma, a much more common salivary gland tumor that is also circumscribed/encapsulated and may also give rise to apocrine intraductal proliferations. However, pleomorphic adenoma lacks acini and shows at least focal well-developed chondromyxoid stroma, a feature that is consistently absent in SPA. The tumors are molecularly distinct as well, with pleomorphic adenoma typically harboring fusions involving *PLAG1* or *HMGA2*.[18]

Intercalated duct lesions or adenomas develop predominantly in the parotid gland, frequently in conjunction with a basal cell adenoma, and are unencapsulated proliferations of intercalated ducts without significant stroma, blending with adjacent acinar cells, and showing few myoepithelial cells. The acinar cells frequently contain large, brightly hypereosinophilic cytoplasmic granules, similar to SPA. However, intercalated duct lesions/adenoma are usually a single, uniform population of cells.[19]

The presence of abnormal, disorganized serous acini within SPA raises the possibility of acinic cell carcinoma. Indeed, the presence of acinar differentiation in a salivary gland tumor is

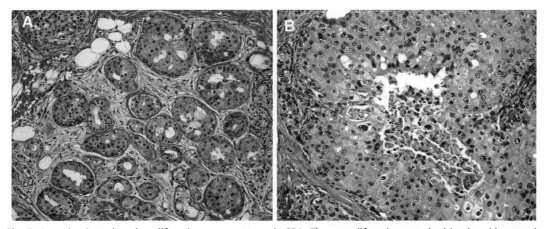

Fig. 7. Apocrine intraductal proliferations are common in SPA. These proliferations can be bland and low grade (*A*) or overtly high grade (*B*).

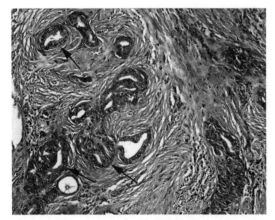

Fig. 8. Highly sclerotic areas of SPA can mimic an invasive carcinoma component. However, close inspection reveals a rim of small, compressed myoepithelial cells (*arrows*) around the glands, confirming that they are still intraductal.

usually diagnostic for acinic cell carcinoma. Showing the presence of myoepithelial cells by immunohistochemistry effectively excludes acinic cell carcinoma. Acinic cell carcinoma usually harbors *NR4A3* rearrangements and shows NR4A3 immunostaining, findings that would be absent in SPA.[20]

In cases of SPA with an apocrine intraductal component, salivary duct carcinoma may be considered. Immunostains for androgen receptor or gross cystic disease fluid protein (GCDFP)-15 are not helpful in distinguishing them, because apocrine elements of any tumor are uniformly positive for these markers. The intraductal elements of SPA, although very similar to salivary duct carcinoma, are entirely surrounded by myoepithelial cells, which can be demonstrated by immunohistochemistry. Moreover, the ductal elements of SPA are associated with other, benign ducts and acini, not seen in salivary duct carcinoma.

Box 1
Key pathologic features of sclerosing polycystic adenoma

- SPA is well circumscribed or encapsulated and often has large cysts

- Proliferative ducts, myoepithelial cells, and acini are present in SPA

- The presence of large, hypereosinophilic cytoplasmic granules is characteristic

- Most, but not all, cases show apocrine metaplasia and intraductal apocrine proliferations that are similar to intraductal carcinoma

---

As mentioned earlier, the apocrine intraductal proliferations seen in many SPAs are, by themselves, indistinguishable from the apocrine variant of intraductal carcinoma. In addition, next-generation sequencing has shown that these 2 tumors are very similar at the molecular level.[21] The additional proliferative ductules and altered acini seen in SPA are not present in pure intraductal carcinoma. Admittedly, the difference between these 2 lesions is not practically important, because they both behave in a benign manner in the absence of stromal invasion.

DIAGNOSIS

Most cases of SPA can be diagnosed based on morphologic features alone:

1. Well-circumscribed lesion with fibrosis and cystic changes.
2. Mixture of ducts, myoepithelial cells, and acini. The myoepithelial cell component may be indistinct and can be highlighted with immunostains for p40, S100 protein, calponin, etc.
3. Large, brightly hypereosinophilic cytoplasmic granules.
4. Ducts with apocrine metaplasia or intraductal carcinoma.

While the recent molecular features of SPA (ie, PI3 kinase pathway mutations and *PTEN* loss) are certainly interesting for classification purposes, they do not a have practical diagnostic role.

PROGNOSIS/TREATMENT

SPA is treated by surgical excision alone. It is not capable of metastasis, but it has been reported to recur in approximately 10% of cases, perhaps because of incomplete excision and persistence.[1,2,5–8,11,12] A single reported case transformed into invasive carcinoma after multiple recurrences over decades.[10]

SUMMARY

SPA is a rare salivary gland lesion that has an unusual constellation of histologic features that may be confused with a variety of reactive conditions, benign neoplasms, and malignant tumors. SPA is characterized by a circumscribed border, fibrosis, cystic changes, hypereosinophilic granules, and a mixture of cell types with frequent intraductal apocrine neoplasia. Even with markedly pleomorphic intraductal cells, SPA is benign and only occasionally recurs after surgical excision. Although originally thought to

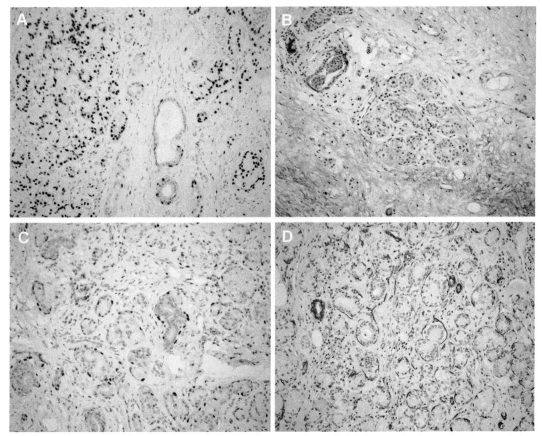

Fig. 9. In SPA, each cellular component has its expected immunoprofile: small ductules, acini, and myoepithelial cells are positive for SOX10 (*A*); acini are positive, albeit often weakly, for DOG1 in a luminal pattern (*B*); and myoepithelial cells are positive for p40 (*C*) and SMA (*D*).

be a nonneoplastic process, recent molecular evidence of clonality and PI3 kinase mutations has established it as a neoplasm.

CLINICS CARE POINTS

- SPA is a benign neoplasm with a mutational profile that is similar to apocrine intraductal carcinoma and salivary duct carcinoma.

- SPA is made up of acini, myoepithelial cells, and ducts that often become cystic and apocrine.

- Large, hypereosinophilic cytoplasmic granules are a helpful histologic clue for SPA.

- Intraductal proliferations are common in SPA, but have no bearing on its nearly uniform benign behavior.

DISCLOSURE

The authors have nothing to disclose.

REFERENCES

1. Smith BC, Ellis GL, Slater LJ, et al. Sclerosing polycystic adenosis of major salivary glands. A clinicopathologic analysis of nine cases. Am J Surg Pathol 1996;20(2):161–70.
2. Seethala R, Gnepp DR, Skalova A, et al. Sclerosing polycystic adenosis. In: el-Naggar AK, Chan JKC, Grandis JR, et al, editors. WHO classification of head and neck tumours. Lyon (France): IARC Press; 2017. p. 195.
3. Skalova A, Gnepp DR, Lewis JS Jr, et al. Newly Described Entities in Salivary Gland Pathology. Am J Surg Pathol 2017;41(8):e33–47.
4. Bishop JA, Gagan J, Baumhoer D, et al. Sclerosing Polycystic "Adenosis" of Salivary Glands: A Neoplasm Characterized by PI3K Pathway Alterations More Correctly Named Sclerosing Polycystic Adenoma. Head Neck Pathol 2019;14(3):630–6.

5. Skalova A, Michal M, Simpson RH, et al. Sclerosing polycystic adenosis of parotid gland with dysplasia and ductal carcinoma in situ. Report of three cases with immunohistochemical and ultrastructural examination. Virchows Arch 2002;440(1):29–35.

6. Skalova A, Gnepp DR, Simpson RH, et al. Clonal nature of sclerosing polycystic adenosis of salivary glands demonstrated by using the polymorphism of the human androgen receptor (HUMARA) locus as a marker. Am J Surg Pathol 2006;30(8):939–44.

7. Gnepp DR, Wang LJ, Brandwein-Gensler M, et al. Sclerosing polycystic adenosis of the salivary gland: a report of 16 cases. Am J Surg Pathol 2006;30(2):154–64.

8. Petersson F. Sclerosing polycystic adenosis of salivary glands: a review with some emphasis on intraductal epithelial proliferations. Head Neck Pathol 2013;7(Suppl 1):S97–106.

9. Su A, Bhuta SM, Berke GS, et al. A unique case of sclerosing polycystic adenosis of the sinonasal tract. Hum Pathol 2013;44(9):1937–40.

10. Canas Marques R, Felix A. Invasive carcinoma arising from sclerosing polycystic adenosis of the salivary gland. Virchows Arch 2014;464(5):621–5.

11. Gnepp DR. Salivary gland tumor "wishes" to add to the next WHO Tumor Classification: sclerosing polycystic adenosis, mammary analogue secretory carcinoma, cribriform adenocarcinoma of the tongue and other sites, and mucinous variant of myoepithelioma. Head Neck Pathol 2014;8(1):42–9.

12. Mokhtari S, Atarbashi Moghadam S, Mirafsharieh A. Sclerosing polycystic adenosis of the retromolar pad area: a case report. Case Rep Pathol 2014;2014:982432.

13. Park IH, Hong SM, Choi H, et al. Sclerosing polycystic adenosis of the nasal septum: the risk of misdiagnosis. Clin Exp Otorhinolaryngol 2013;6(2):107–9.

14. Pfeiffer ML, Yin VT, Bell D, et al. Sclerosing polycystic adenosis of the lacrimal gland. Ophthalmology 2013;120(4):873–873.e1.

15. Petersson F, Tan PH, Hwang JS. Sclerosing polycystic adenosis of the parotid gland: report of a bifocal, paucicystic variant with ductal carcinoma in situ and pronounced stromal distortion mimicking invasive carcinoma. Head Neck Pathol 2011;5(2):188–92.

16. Kumar KA, Mahadesh J, Setty S. Dysgenetic polycystic disease of the parotid gland: Report of a case and review of the literature. J Oral Maxillofac Pathol 2013;17(2):248–52.

17. Agaimy A. Fat-containing salivary gland tumors: a review. Head Neck Pathol 2013;7(Suppl 1):S90–6.

18. Katabi N, Xu B, Jungbluth AA, et al. PLAG1 immunohistochemistry is a sensitive marker for pleomorphic adenoma: a comparative study with PLAG1 genetic abnormalities. Histopathology 2018;72(2):285–93.

19. Weinreb I, Seethala RR, Hunt JL, et al. Intercalated duct lesions of salivary gland: a morphologic spectrum from hyperplasia to adenoma. Am J Surg Pathol 2009;33(9):1322–9.

20. Haller F, Skalova A, Ihrler S, et al. Nuclear NR4A3 Immunostaining is a Specific and Sensitive Novel Marker for Acinic Cell Carcinoma of the Salivary Glands. Am J Surg Pathol 2019;43(9):1264–72.

21. Bishop JA, Gagan J, Krane JF, et al. Low-grade Apocrine Intraductal Carcinoma: Expanding the Morphologic and Molecular Spectrum of an Enigmatic Salivary Gland Tumor. Head Neck Pathol 2020;14(4):869–75.

Basal Cell Adenoma and Basal Cell Adenocarcinoma

Robert A. Robinson, MD, PhD

KEYWORDS

- Basal cell adenoma • Basal cell adenocarcinoma • Salivary gland tumors

Key points

- Basal cell adenoma (BCA) and basal cell adenocarcinoma (BCAC) are uncommon biphasic salivary gland tumors having morphologic similarities to other biphasic salivary gland neoplasms with differentiation toward the intercalated ducts of the salivary gland.
- BCA and BCAC show 4 patterns: tubular, trabecular, solid, and membranous.
- BCA are benign neoplasms, but membranous BCA have a high recurrence rate.
- BCAC are low-grade malignant tumors and are separated from BCA primarily on their invasive properties.
- BCA and BCAC are best diagnosed using routine hematoxylin and eosin sections.

ABSTRACT

Basal cell adenoma (BCA) and basal cell adenocarcinoma (BCAC) are uncommon biphasic salivary gland tumors having morphologic similarities to other biphasic salivary gland neoplasms having differentiation toward the intercalated ducts of the salivary gland. Both tumors show mixtures of trabecular, tubular, solid, and membranous solid patterns. BCAC is separated from BCA primarily by the presence of invasion in the former. The diagnosis of BCA and BCAC is best carried out with hematoxylin and eosin–stained sections and careful attention to detail of tumors in the differential diagnosis, including adenoid cystic carcinoma, pleomorphic adenoma, and epithelial myoepithelial carcinoma.

OVERVIEW

Basal cell adenoma (BCA) and basal cell adenocarcinoma (BCAC) are uncommon salivary gland tumors. They are among several biphasic salivary gland neoplasms with varying degrees of morphologic similarity composed of small basaloid cells with inner (luminal) ductal epithelial cells and outer (abluminal) basal/myoepithelial cells. Their recognition is important to separate them from these similar appearing tumors that have differing biologic behavior.

CLINICAL FINDINGS

BCA and BCAC are not common, with BCA comprising 5% to 6% of benign salivary gland tumors and BCAC comprising 1% to 3% of malignant salivary gland tumors. Gender balance in each shows a near equal proportion, and both occur over a wide age range, most often in the sixth to seventh decade.[1–5]

Both BCA and BCAC may occur in major or minor salivary glands, but the parotid gland is the most common site.[4,5] The next most common site is the submandibular gland followed by the sublingual gland and then the minor salivary glands in the head and neck, including buccal mucosa, palate, tongue, and even more rare sites, such as the parapharynx.[6–8] Several investigators have noted that a significant percentage of BCACs arise from preexisting BCAs.[5,9]

Department of Pathology, University of Iowa, University of Iowa Carver College of Medicine, 5238 H Roy Carver Pavilion, 200 Hawkins Drive, Iowa City, IA 52242, USA
E-mail address: robert-a-robinson@uiowa.edu

Surgical Pathology 14 (2021) 25–42
https://doi.org/10.1016/j.path.2020.09.005
1875-9181/21/© 2020 Elsevier Inc. All rights reserved.

surgpath.theclinics.com

GROSS FEATURES

BCAs commonly range in size from 0.5 to 5 cm, but most are 2 to 2.5 cm (**Box 1**).[1,4] They are generally present as a single nodule, but membranous patterned BCAs are noted to show multinodular growth. Tumors are typically well circumscribed, and many are encapsulated, particularly in the major glands. When arising in minor glands, a capsule may not be seen, but the tumor is always circumscribed. Cystic change, a common feature microscopically, may be observed grossly.

BCAC are incompletely circumscribed, and if encapsulated, can show invasive areas pushing through the capsule. They may also show cystic change. BCAC are noted as being larger on average than BCA. In a single-institutional study, 29 tumors ranged in size from 0.9 to 8.5 cm with a mean of 2.9 cm.[1]

MICROSCOPIC FEATURES

MICROSCOPIC FEATURES OF BASAL CELL ADENOMA

BCA demonstrates the bilayering of cells mimicking what is observed in intercalated and striated ducts of the salivary gland unit[10] (**Box 2**).

The low-power view of BCA reveals a circumscribed neoplasm, and in the major glands, the tumor is often encapsulated (**Fig. 1**). Despite a relatively low-power appearance of basaloid monomorphous tumor cells, there is a biphasic mix of cellular differentiation, including ductal (luminal) and basal and myoepithelial (abluminal) cells, which can be elucidated at higher magnification with routine staining.[4] Luminal cells are characterized by small nearly cuboidal cells surrounding an abluminal layer of slightly larger cells with paler cytoplasm, which is itself overlayered with smaller more hyperchromatic myoepithelial cells.[10]

The neoplastic cells are arranged in trabecular, tubular, solid, and membranous patterns with mixtures of these patterns common in most tumors. These nests are separated from each other by usually loose collagen strands. The periphery of the nests shows a palisaded arrangement. The trabecular pattern has long columns of basaloid cells, usually 2 to 5 cells thick (**Fig. 2**). The tubular pattern shows small tubular structures lined by epithelial cells in which the tubules are connected in long anastomosing cords (**Fig. 3**). Solid patterned tumors are characterized by packs of closely approximated basaloid cells in nests or islands (**Fig. 4**). A distinctive subtype morphology that is shared with dermal

Fig. 1. BCA with a rounded fibrous capsule separating it from the surrounding parotid gland (hematoxylin and eosin, original magnification X100).

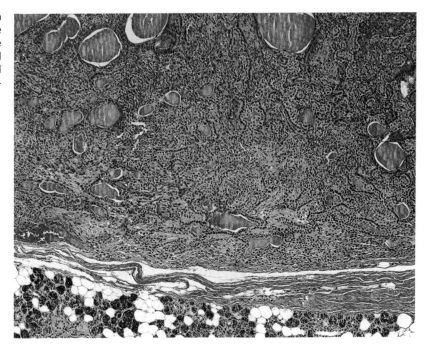

Fig. 1. BCA with a rounded fibrous capsule separating it from the surrounding parotid gland (hematoxylin and eosin, original magnification X100).

cylindromas is one termed membranous (dermal analogue).[11] Membranous patterns show dense acellular hyaline basement membrane-like material surrounding nests of basaloid cells as well as being deposited between cells (**Fig. 5**). To qualify as a membranous BCA, the tumor should have a predominance of the membranous pattern, as small amounts of hyaline material

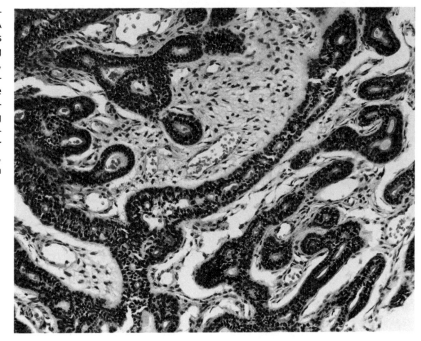

Fig. 2. BCA with trabecular pattern. BCA frequently show patterns with long anastomosing trabeculae. Commonly, small dilatations are present in the center of the trabeculae, forming lumens and delineating the luminal and abluminal aspects of the tumor (hematoxylin and eosin, original magnification X200).

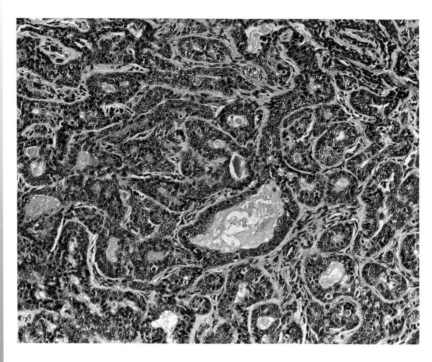

Fig. 3. BCA with tubular pattern. This BCA is predominantly composed of tubular structures (hematoxylin and eosin, original magnification X200).

may be seen admixed in other patterns. The membranous patterned tumors have a much greater propensity to recur, and it is important to separate them from the other patterns seen in BCA. BCA can have areas of overt squamous differentiation (**Fig. 6**). Some BCA show intervening spindled stromal cells[12] (**Fig. 7**). Occasionally, a cribriform arrangement may be seen, but if present, it is focal and lacks a crisp punched-out appearance.

Fig.4. BCA, solid pattern. BCA is seen with completely solid growth pattern in this field (hematoxylin and eosin, original magnification X200).

Fig. 5. BCAC, membranous pattern. This BCAC has dense hyaline material between solid islands of tumor as well as between cells; however, no mitotic figures or areas of invasion are seen in this image. Because both BCA and BCAC may all show identical trabecular, solid, tubular, and membranous patterns, close observation for the presence of invasion and mitotic figures is required to exclude BCAC (hematoxylin and eosin, original magnification X200).

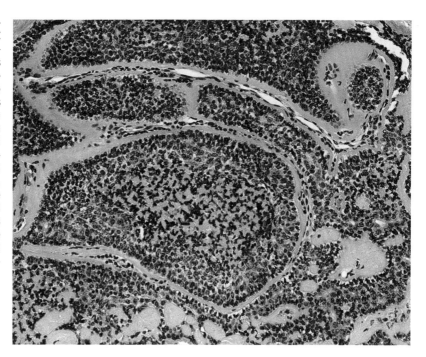

MICROSCOPIC FEATURES OF BASAL CELL ADENOCARCINOMA

BCAC is a near cytologic mimic of BCA with mixtures of tubular, trabecular, solid, and membranous patterns, with most having a solid pattern.[1,4] The key finding in separating BCA and BCAC is an invasive growth pattern, which may be seen as an irregular interface with the surrounding tissues or as a rounded mass of cells with

Fig.6. Squamous changes may be seen in BCA or BCAC, as present in this BCA, where the luminal cells in a trabecula have become larger and eosinophilic (hematoxylin and eosin, original magnification X200).

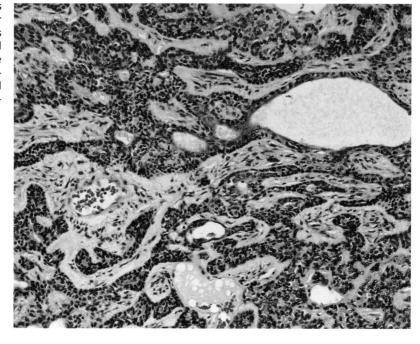

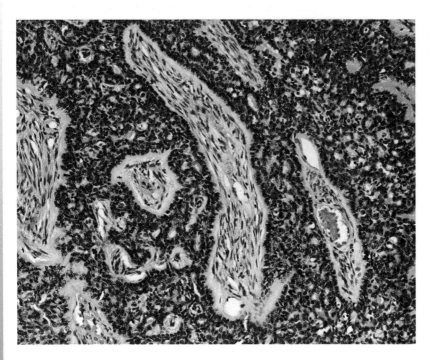

Fig. 7. The intervening stroma of BCA or BCAC may show spindled cells (hematoxylin and eosin, original magnification X400).

destructive characteristics, pushing or splitting apart normal salivary gland parenchyma or adipose tissue. The invasive foci may take a rounded or nodular appearance (**Fig. 8**). Perineural invasion may also be seen but is not present in all cases.[1,6]

The finding of mitotic figures is also useful in separation of BCA and BCAC, with the latter often showing at least some mitotic figures (**Fig. 9**). However, even in BCAC mitoses are rarely abundant. Most studies suggest that more than 3 to 4

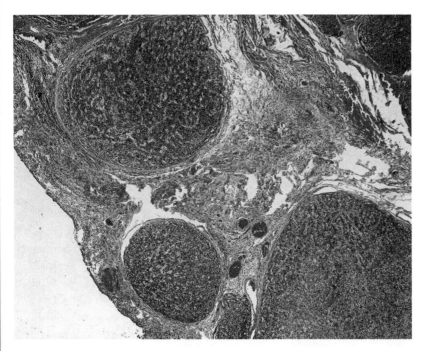

Fig. 8. An invasive front of BCAC is seen as tumor nodules invading the surrounding fibrous tissue (hematoxylin and eosin, original magnification X40).

Fig. 9. BCAC have mitotic figures, but they may be limited in number (hematoxylin and eosin, original magnification X600).

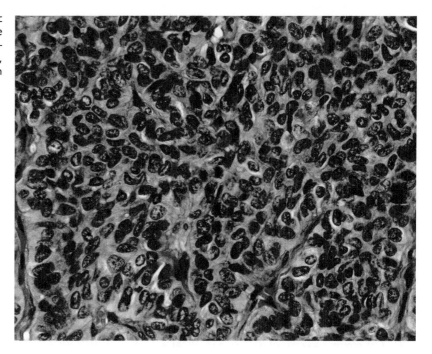

mitoses/high-power field (HPF) correlate with a diagnosis of BCAC over BCA.[1,4,9,13] Although BCACs are considered by most as low grade and lack severe atypia and necrosis, some reports have noted necrosis and vascular invasion more commonly.[13]

BASALOID BIPHASIC SALIVARY GLAND TUMORS IN THE DIFFERENTIAL DIAGNOSIS OF BASAL CELL ADENOMA AND BASAL CELL ADENOCARCINOMA

Adenoid cystic carcinoma (ACC), epithelial myoepithelial carcinoma (EMC), and cellular pleomorphic adenoma (PA) are basaloid tumors with morphologic similarities to BCA and BCAC, which have a biphasic cellular arrangement (**Box 3**). Morphologic clues on hematoxylin and eosin staining usually suffice to separate these neoplasms, and although some limited immunohistochemical studies can more strongly point to some of these entities over others, none are foolproof, owing to similar cell cytologic differentiation being similar between the members of this group. Molecular distinction (see later discussion) can help in some cases when specific molecular abnormalities are detected.

BASAL CELL ADENOMA/BASAL CELL ADENOCARCINOMA VERSUS ADENOID CYSTIC CARCINOMA

Separation of ACC from BCA and BCAC is accomplished using architectural and cytologic criteria. ACC is characterized by tubular, cribriform, and solid patterns. The solid variant of ACC, a tumor that shows abundant solid areas of with a reduced percentage of tubular or cribriform patterns overall, is the most likely to be confused with a solid pattern BCA or BCAC.[14,15] However, even solid ACC has some classic cribriform patterns that have small cleared areas with an appearance of a round, cleanly punched-out area filled with a hyaline material (**Fig. 10**). The nuclei of ACC are angular rather than rounded, and the cell arrangements are not palisaded. ACC has an infiltrative border as small cells at low power, whereas BCA has a rounded border (**Fig. 11**). Most BCAC also have rounded borders, even if invasive, although these tumors can show individual cell infiltration from the periphery. BCA and BCAC have nested cells with peripheral palisaded patterns and a distinct arrangement of cells with paler cytoplasm in the center of the nests with smaller and darker cells at the periphery. This peripheral patterning can be useful in separating BCA from other basaloid lesions, such as ACC. Stromal spindled areas

> **Box 3**
> **Key points in differential diagnosis of basal cell adenoma and basal cell adenocarcinoma**
>
> - Morphology seen on routine H&E staining is most useful and reliable.
> - Immunohistochemical staining can help in differentiating some situations, but staining overlap with other bilayered salivary gland tumors can be problematic.
> - ACC usually shows classic cribriform patterns with distinct punched out spaces surrounded by small cells with minimal cytoplasm and hyperchromatic, often angular nuclei, findings uncommon in BCA or BCAC.
> - In separation from PA, BCA or BCAC does not display myxoid/chondromyxoid, mucoid, or cartilaginous areas as seen in PA, nor do their component cells display prominent plasmacytoid cells.
> - BCA and BCAC have sharp delineation of the epithelial/myoepithelial cell components from the stroma, while PA, even though containing similar cellular components, shows a blending with the background stroma.
> - EMC, a bilayered malignant salivary gland tumor, often has clear cells as its abluminal layer, a finding very unusual for BCA or BCAC.
> - Limited biopsy material may make the separation of these entities difficult.

as seen in some BCA and BCAC are not present in ACC. Cribriform variants of BCAs and BCACs have been described as well, but the acellular spaces in this pattern often have a dense pink hyaline material often containing embedded cells or vascular cores, findings not seen in ACC (**Fig. 12**). Perineural invasion is a common finding in ACC that may be seen in BCACs as well, although the perineural invasion in ACC is usually much more extensive compared with BCAC.

Although there are morphologic differences between BCA/BCAC and ACC, limited biopsies may hinder the distinction.

BASAL CELL ADENOMA/BASAL CELL ADENOCARCINOMA VERSUS PLEOMORPHIC ADENOMA

Although most PAs do not cause difficulty in the differential diagnosis, those that are cellular or in

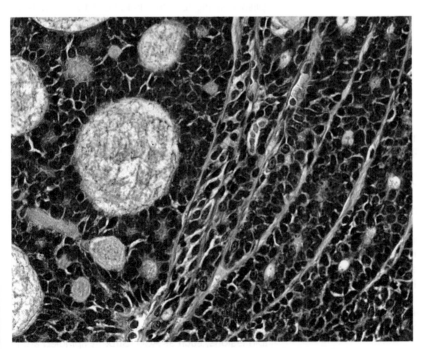

Fig. 10. ACC with adjoining cribriform and tubular components. The cribriform luminal structures are cleanly and uniformly "punched out" and are not seen to this degree in the cribriform patterns in BCA or BCAC (hematoxylin and eosin, original magnification X600).

Fig. 11. BCA with a cribriform pattern. A cribriform pattern can suggest ACC in either BCA or BCAC. Unlike ACC, the pattern present has less well-defined, more irregular structural shapes. In some of the central areas, there are individual cells or small vessels, a finding not seen in ACC (hematoxylin and eosin, original magnification X200).

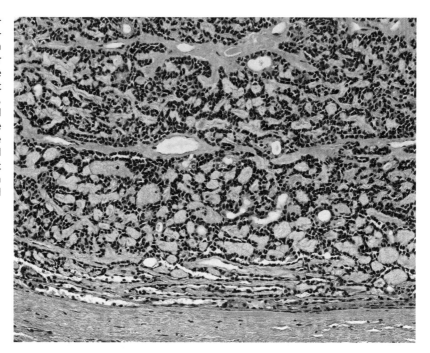

cases where a limited amount of material is available can cause some problems in separation. BCA or BCAC does not display myxoid/chondromyxoid, mucoid, or cartilaginous areas as seen in PA, nor do their component cells display a plasmacytoid or have myoepithelial clear cells[16] (**Fig. 13**). Both BCA and BCAC may show squamous change, but that finding is much more common in PA. BCA and BCAC have sharp delineation of the epithelial/myoepithelial cell components

Fig. 12. BCA with hyaline cores in a cribriform pattern show some resemblance to that of ACC. These have centrally placed cells in some cores, a finding not seen in ACC (hematoxylin and eosin, original magnification X600).

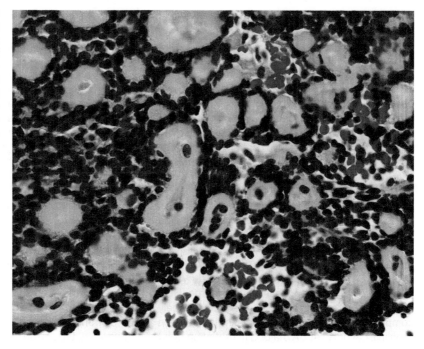

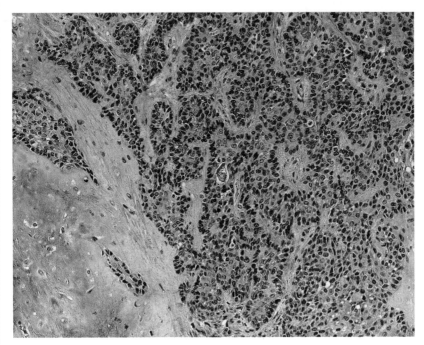

Fig. 13. The epithelial cells in this PA are arranged in a trabecular pattern, where a luminal and abluminal pattern can be discerned, very similar to that of BCA with which it can be confused. Foci of chondromyxoid areas in PA help separate the two (hematoxylin and eosin, original magnification X200).

from the stroma, whereas PA, even though containing similar cellular components, show a blending with the background stroma. The distinct stromal cells sometimes seen in BCA and BCAC are not seen in PA.

BASAL CELL ADENOMA/BASAL CELL ADENOCARCINOMA VERSUS EPITHELIAL MYOEPITHELIAL CARCINOMA

EMCs are most commonly seen in the major glands, particularly the parotid and submandibular gland and sometimes seen in the minor glands. They are mostly low-grade tumors, but higher-grade tumors are described. A striking finding in many EMC is its multinodular but invasive growth pattern, although that is a pattern sometimes shared with BCAC.[17] The classic pattern of EMC is a malignant salivary gland tumor composed of a biphasic arrangement of inner eosinophilic luminal ductal cells and outer clear myoepithelial cells.[18,19] EMC can show a much more diverse morphologic appearance with spindled, clear, or oncocytic differentiation and occasionally with marked atypia, findings not seen in BCA or BCAC.[20] EMC frequently show a myxoid-hyaline stroma, a finding also shared with some BCA and BCAC, but an abluminal layer that is largely composed cells with clear cytoplasm is not often seen in BCA or BCAC. A major differentiating point

between EMC and BCA is the frequent perineural invasion present in EMC, a feature not seen in BCA. BCAC may also exhibit perineural invasion, but it is not common.

DIAGNOSIS

Immunohistochemistry is rarely needed to establish a diagnosis of BCA or BCAC in the separation of either from basaloid salivary gland neoplasms if the tumor is completely excised. In the case of limited material, immunohistochemical studies may help point to the correct diagnosis (**Box 4**).

Pan-cytokeratin expression is present in nearly all tumors, with greatest intensity in the luminal cells compared with abluminal, the latter of which can be variable in intensity. Overall, low-molecular-weight keratins are more strongly expressed in areas with luminal differentiation[21–24] (**Fig. 14**). The luminal cell types may also show some S100 staining as well as positivity for EMA and even CEA.

As opposed to luminal cells, the abluminal basal/myoepithelial cells in BCA and BCAC show strong staining with high-molecular-weight keratins, such as 34betaE12, CK14, and CK5, as well as other markers, such as p63 and p40[22,25,26] (**Figs. 15** and **16**). These cells are further positive for calponin, muscle-specific actin, alpha smooth muscle actin, S100, and vimentin (**Fig. 17**).

> **Box 4**
> **Key points of diagnosis**
>
> - Immunohistochemistry is rarely needed to establish a diagnosis of BCA or BCAC in the separation of either from basaloid salivary gland neoplasms when the entire tumor is excised.
>
> - BCA/BCAC show epithelial, basal, and myoepithelial differentiation, limiting the markers that can be useful in separating basaloid salivary gland neoplasms, as the common tumors in the differential diagnosis have the same fundamental cellular makeup.
>
> - Beta-catenin expression may be helpful in the diagnosis when used in conjunction with routine hematoxylin and eosin staining.
>
> - Caution should be used in interpreting immunohistochemical expression of beta-catenin for separation of BCA or BCAC from other basaloid neoplasms in the differential diagnosis with definitive diagnosis requiring careful histologic assessment with hematoxylin and eosin stain.

Besides having occasional luminal as well as some abluminal cells expression, S100 is also strongly expressed in the spindled stromal type cells seen in the BCA pattern described as trabecular-tubular. S100 in a stromal staining pattern can be useful when present, as ACC and EMC do not show this.[22]

Studies have investigated beta-catenin to help separate BCA and BCAC from other basaloid salivary gland neoplasms in the differential diagnosis[27–29] (**Fig. 18**). Staining is generally patchy and present mostly in the basaloid cells, but the S100-positive stromal cells also stain. Beta-catenin has been shown in several studies not to be expressed or expressed in only limited numbers of cases of ACC, EMC or PA.[27,29–32] or Caution should be used in relying solely on immunohistochemical expression of beta-catenin for absolute separation of BCA or BCAC from other basaloid neoplasms in the differential diagnosis. Most but not all studies have reported the beta-catenin expression as nuclear staining in BCA and BCAC, as it can be seen in the membrane and cytoplasm in other tumors in the differential.[33–35]

Ki67 staining is variable in BCA and BCAC but with much higher values in BCAC compared with BCA.[1,13,22] In 1 series, the average proliferation

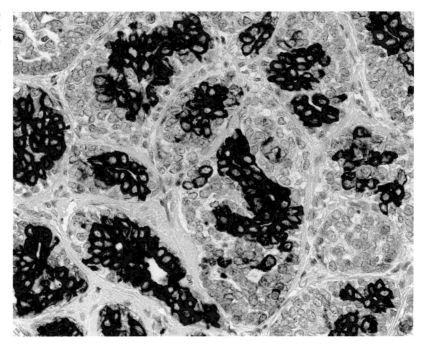

Fig. 14. CK7 stains the luminal aspect of this BCA (original magnification X400).

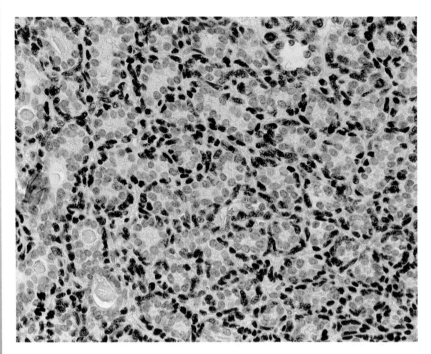

Fig. 15. The abluminal cells are clearly seen enhanced by p63 staining in this tubular pattern BCA (original magnification X400).

index was 3.3% and 15.5% for BCA and BCAC, respectively.[1] Thus, a low Ki67 is associated with BCA and mitigates against BCAC, ACC, and EMC. A high Ki67 does not help in the separation of BCAC and ACC and EMC.

ACC is associated with a recurrent chromosomal translocation t(6;9)(q22-23;p23-24) in which an *MYB* and *NFIB* fusion results and can be demonstrated in more than half of cases. MYB protein expression has been used to support a diagnosis of ACC. Although MYB

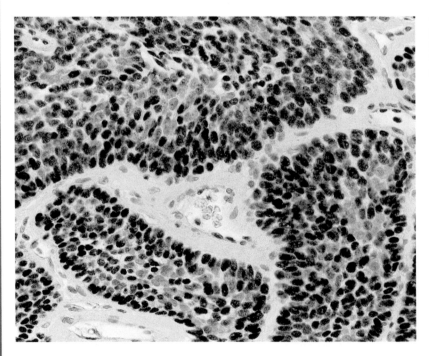

Fig. 16. A solid pattern BCAC reveals p63 staining in abluminal locations (original magnification X400).

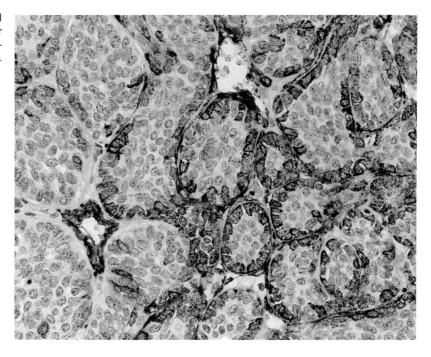

Fig. 17. The abluminal cells are positive for SMSA in this BCAC (original magnification X400).

immunohistochemical staining is often seen in ACC, its expression has been noted in BCA and BCAC[36,37] (**Fig. 19**).

Other antibodies used to differentiate salivary gland neoplasms, including CD117, DOG1, and GFAP, are seen to be variably expressed in some BCA and BCAC.[21,38,39] PLAG1, commonly expressed in PA, has been reported in BCAC.[40] Although the SRY-related HMG-box 10 (Sox 10) is a marker for neural crest–derived cells, it is seen in myoepithelial cells of multiple organs. CD117, DOG1, GFAP, PLAG1 and Sox 10 also encompass a wide variety of salivary gland neoplasms, including BCA, BCAC, PA, ACC, and

Fig. 18. Beta-catenin is present in this trabecular patterned BCA, where it is localized mostly in the abluminal cells (original magnification X400).

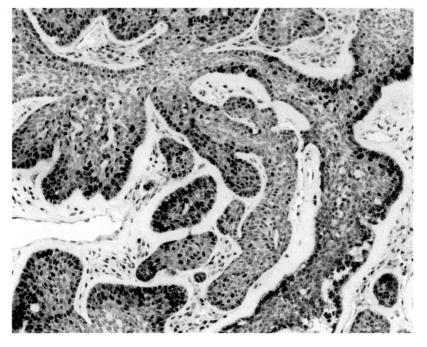

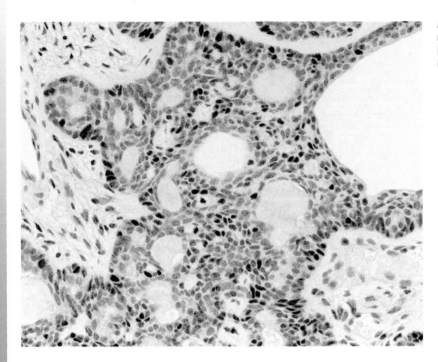

Fig. 19. Immunohistochemical staining with Myb is present in a BCA (original magnification X400).

EMC.[41] p53 overexpression has been reported in both BCA and BCAC but also in other salivary gland tumors, rendering its use limited.[17]

MOLECULAR PATHOLOGY FINDINGS IN BASAL CELL ADENOMA AND BASAL CELL ADENOCARCINOMA

Studies of pathology findings at the molecular level have given way to increasing knowledge of BCAs and BCACs (Box 5). In most instances, these studies have led back to connections to the complex aspects of salivary gland organogenesis. Many of the genes involved in the cross-talk network of signaling proteins orchestrating epithelial and mesenchymal involvement in developing acini and ducts in a stromal matrix are seen to be involved in salivary gland tumor development as well.[42–44]

Two of the most frequently studied genes in BCA and BCAC are *CTNNB1*, which codes for beta-catenin, and *CYLD*, which encodes a deubiquitinating enzyme, CYLD. These genes, as well as many others, are intricately involved in Wnt pathways. Normally, beta-catenin is usually held in E-cadherin adherens junctions, and free beta-catenin is depleted by ubiquitin-mediated degradation. However, free beta-catenin can accumulate because of *CTNNB1* mutations or losses of APC or Axin function. When normal degradation of cytoplasmic beta-catenin is arrested, there can be subsequent movement of beta-catenin to the nucleus, where it can activate other target genes, transcription alone or in tandem with other factors, such as transcription factor T-cell factor/lymphoid enhancer factor.[45] These factors can then impact the expression of c-Myc and cyclin D1. *CYLD*, which modifies several signaling proteins by removal of ubiquitin. is thought to be a negative regulator that sits upstream of the Wnt/beta-catenin pathway, as inhibition of *CYLD* enhances Wnt-induced beta-catenin stabilization.[45–47]

Box 5
Key points of molecular pathology findings in basal cell adenoma and basal cell adenocarcinoma

- BCA shows frequent CTNNB-1 alterations but not all tumors have mutations.
- Both BCA and BCAC show CYLD mutations in some but not all tumors.
- PIK3CA mutations are seen in BCAC in some but not all tumors.

Numerous studies have shown the involvement of the beta-catenin gene in BCAs with nuclear beta-catenin expression in most BCA and with activating mutations of *CTNNB1* seen in up to half the cases.[27,28,30,48] *CTNNB1* mutations have been reported to be associated with a predominance of a tubular or tubulotrabecular patterns as opposed to solid, trabecular, or cribriform patterns.[28] Of note, many studies that have also investigated *CTTNB1* gene abnormalities and have found beta-catenin is often expressed in the nucleus without concomitant gene abnormality. Although *CTNNB1* activating mutations are present in BCA, only rare reports of these mutations exist in BCAC, a tumor that also frequently shows beta-catenin nuclear expression. It is presumed other mechanisms account for the nuclear expression in non-*CTNNB1* mutated tumors. Although mutations in *CTNNB1*, *AXIN*, or *APC* give rise to nuclear beta-catenin accumulation, these mutations have been reported in ACC and PA.[33,49] However, most studies show that ACC have much lower incidence of *CTNNB1* mutations than BCA, with some reports showing no mutations.[29] PA demonstrates *CTNNB1-PLAG1* fusions, with *CTNNB1* being one of the most common gene partners in PA. This translocation, t(3;8)(p21;q12), is one in which *PLAG1*, a zinc-finger gene, is activated by a *CTNNB1* promoter.[50,51] However, it is likely that the *CTNNB1* gene is not directly related to the tumor development of PA in these cases.[35]

CYLD gene is a tumor suppressor gene located on chromosome 16q12-q13 and is associated with Brooke-Spiegler syndrome, an inherited autosomal dominant disease with numerous associated cutaneous adnexal tumors, including cylindroma, spiradenoma, and trichoepithelioma. Although BCA occur in this syndrome, they only occur in a minority of patients.[52] Most CYLD mutations occurring in BCA or BCAC do so outside of syndromic conditions. In 1 study, multiple missense mutations were found in 36% of BCA and 29% of BCAC with the mutations in BCA occurring in differing domains than the BCAC.[53]

PIK3CA functions as an oncogene and is situated on chromosome 3q26, which encodes the p110 alpha subunit of class IA phosphatidylinositol 3-kinase, a subunit critical for the control of protein synthesis, angiogenesis, and cellular proliferation through the PI3K/Akt pathway. Mutations of the gene have been described in many tumors, including BCAC but not BCA.[1,27] However, mutations have been described in other salivary gland basaloid neoplasms, such as ACC as well as nonbasaloid salivary gland tumors, including salivary duct carcinoma and mucoepidermoid carcinoma.[54,55] *PIK3CA* has been thought to be a potential gene for targeted therapy.

PROGNOSIS

BASAL CELL ADENOMA

The prognosis of BCA is good with complete conservative excision representing adequate therapy for BCA. However, the membranous pattern is associated with recurrences.[1,2] The rate of recurrence of membranous BCA is generally reported to be 25%, and one of the reasons for its recurrence is suggested to be its frequent multinodularity.[1,5] Some investigators have suggested that BCA can be the precursor to BCAC. Whether these other morphologies arose subsequently or concurrently is not always clear.

BASAL CELL ADENOCARCINOMA

BCAC is generally considered a low-grade malignancy with deaths owing to tumor uncommonly occurring.[4,5] Because of the rarity of BCAC, there are limited data on the natural history of BCAC, including its metastatic potential. Percentages of recurrence, local, and distant metastases vary by report. Recurrence rates have been reported from 15% to 50%, with most reported rates of approximately 30%. Less than 10% develop cervical lymph node metastases, and less than 5% develop distant metastases and death.[5,13]

SUMMARY

BCA and BCAC are uncommon biphasic salivary gland tumors having morphologic similarities to other biphasic salivary gland neoplasms having differentiation toward the intercalated ducts of the salivary gland. Both tumors show identical architectural patterns of trabecular, tubular, solid, and membranous. The diagnosis of BCA and BCAC is best carried out with hematoxylin and eosin–stained sections and careful attention to detail of tumors in the differential diagnosis, including ACC, PA, and EMC. Many BCA show activating mutations of the *CTNNB1* gene, and *PIK3CA* mutations are seen in BCAC, but these are described in other tumors in the differential diagnosis. BCA is a benign neoplasm, but the membranous pattern has a high recurrence rate. Although BCAC is malignant, it is low grade and generally has a good prognosis.

CLINICS CARE POINTS

- Small biopsies may make histologic distinction impossible when the differential diagnosis includes PA, BCA/BCAC, ACC, and EMC.
- In the dissection and grossing of salivary gland tumors, it is important to include normal or nonneoplastic tissue that contains sections of the tumor, as the separation of BCA from BCAC is highly dependent on whether there is invasion of surrounding normal tissue.
- The sharp delineation of the epithelial/myoepithelial cellular components from the stroma is present in BCA and BCAC, but not in PA, aiding in their separation.
- Careful attention must be given to any significant membranous component in BCA to determine if the tumor is a membranous variant, one in which there is a high recurrence rate.
- Beta-catenin staining, in conjunction with careful evaluation of hematoxylin and eosin–stained sections, can be useful to establish the diagnosis of BCA/BCAC.

DISCLOSURE

The author has nothing to disclose.

REFERENCES

1. Wilson TC, Robinson RA. Basal cell adenocarcinoma and basal cell adenoma of the salivary glands: a clinicopathological review of seventy tumors with comparison of morphologic features and growth control indices. Head Neck Pathol 2015;9:205–13.
2. Tian Z, Li L, Wang L, et al. Salivary gland neoplasms in oral and maxillofacial regions: a 23-year retrospective study of 6982 cases in an Eastern Chinese population. Int J Oral Maxillofac Surg 2010;39(3): 235–42.
3. Ellis G, Wiscovitch J. Basal cell adenocarcinomas of the major salivary glands. Oral Surg Oral Med Oral Pathol 1990;69:461–9.
4. Ellis GL, Auclair PL. Tumors of the salivary glands. Atlas of tumor pathology, 4th series, Fascicle 9. Silver Spring (NM): ARP Press; 2008.
5. Muller S, Barnes L. Basal cell adenocarcinoma of the salivary glands: report of seven cases and review of the literature. Cancer 1996;78(12):2471–7.
6. Fonseca I, Soares J. Basal cell adenocarcinoma of minor salivary and seromucous glands of the head and neck region. Semin Diagn Pathol 1996;13(2): 128–37.
7. Triest W, Fried M, Stanievich J. Membranous basal cell adenoma of the hypopharynx. Arch Otolaryngol 1983;109(11):774–7.
8. Cuthbertson D, Raol N, Hicks J, et al. Minor salivary gland basal cell adenocarcinoma: a systematic review and report of a new case. JAMA Otolaryngol Head Neck Surg 2015;141(3):276–83.
9. Nagao T, Sugano I, Ishid Y, et al. Carcinoma in basal cell adenoma of the parotid gland. Pathol Res Pract 1997;193:171–8.
10. Seethala R. Basaloid/blue salivary gland tumors. Mod Pathol 2017;30:s84–95.
11. Yu G, Ubmuller J, Donath K. Membranous basal cell adenoma of the salivary gland: a clinicopathologic study of 12 cases. Acta Otolaryngol 1998;118(4): 588–93.
12. Ortolani E, Polimeni A, Lauriola L, et al. Basal cell adenoma with S-100 positive stroma: a case report and literature review. Oral Surg Oral Med Oral Pathol Oral Radiol 2016;121:e62–4.
13. Nagao T, Sugano I, Ishida Y, et al. Basal cell adenocarcinoma of the salivary glands: comparison with basal cell adenoma through assessment of cell proliferation, apoptosis, and expression of p53 and bcl-2. Cancer 1998;82(3):439–47.
14. Li B-B, Zhou C-X, Jia S-N. Basal cell adenoma of salivary glands with a focal cribriform pattern: clinicopathologic and immunohistochemical study of 19 cases of a potential pitfall for diagnosis. Ann Diagn Pathol 2014;18:5–9.
15. Zhou Y, Martinez Duarte M, Eleff D, et al. An unusual hybrid salivary gland tumor: molecular analysis informs the potential pathogenesis of this rare neoplasm. Case Rep Pathol 2019;2713234. https://doi.org/10.1155/2019/2713234.
16. Chhieng D, Paulino A. Basaloid tumors of the salivary glands. Ann Diagn Pathol 2002;6:364–72.
17. Seethala R, Barnes E. Rare malignant and benign salivary gland epithelial tumors. Surg Pathol Clin 2011;4(4):1217–72.
18. Di Palma S. Epithelial-myoepithelial carcinoma with co-existing multifocal intercalated duct hyperplasia of the parotid gland. Histopathology 1994;25: 494–6.
19. Corio R, Sciubba J, Brannon R, et al. Epithelial-myoepithelial carcinoma of intercalated duct origin. A clinicopathologic and ultrastructural assessment of sixteen cases. Oral Pathol 1982;53(3):280–7.
20. Bishop J, Westra W. MYB translocation status in salivary gland epithelial-myoepithelial carcinoma: evaluation of classic, variant, and hybrid forms. Am J Surg Pathol 2018;42(3):319–25.
21. Williams S, Ellis G, Auclair P. Immunohistochemical analysis of basal cell adenocarcinoma. Oral Surg Oral Med Oral Pathol 1993;75:64–9.

22. Nagao T, Sato E, Inoue H, et al. Immunohistochemical analysis of salivary gland tumors: application for surgical pathology practice. Acta Histochem Cytochem 2012;45(5):269–82.

23. Ogawa I, Nikai H, Takata T, et al. The cellular composition of basal cell adenoma of the parotid gland: an immunohistochemical analysis. Oral Surg Oral Med Oral Pathol 1990;70:619–26.

24. Ferreiro J. Immunohistochemistry of basal cell adenoma of the major salivary glands. Histopathology 1994;24:539–42.

25. Owosho A, Aguilar C, Seethala R. Comparison of p63 and p40 (ΔNp63) as basal, squamoid and myoepithelial markers in salivary gland tumors. Appl Immunohistochem Mol Morphol 2016;24:501–8.

26. Edwards P, Bhuiya T, Kelsch R. Assessment of p63 expression in the salivary gland neoplasms adenoid cystic carcinoma, polymorphous low-grade adenocarcinoma, and basal cell and canalicular adenomas. Oral Surg Oral Med Oral Pathol Oral Radiol Endod 2004;97(5):613–9.

27. Jo V, Sholl L, Krane J. Distinctive patterns of *CTNNB1* (b-catenin) alterations in salivary gland basal cell adenoma and basal cell adenocarcinoma. Am J Surg Pathol 2016;40(8):1143–50.

28. Lee Y, Huang W, Hsieh M. *CTNNB1*mutations in basal cell adenoma of the salivary gland. J Formos Med Assoc 2018;117(10):894–901.

29. Sato M, Yamamoto H, Hatanaka Y, et al. Wnt/beta-catenin signal alteration and its diagnostic utility in basal cell adenoma and histologically similar tumors of the salivary gland. Pathol Res Pract 2018;214(4):586–92.

30. Kawahara A, Harada H, Abe H, et al. Nuclear beta catenin expression in basal cell adenomas of salivary gland. J Oral Pathol Med 2011;40(6):460–6.

31. do Prado R, Cardoso C, Consolaro A, et al. Nuclear beta catenin in basal cell adenomas. Int J Surg Pathol 2007;15(2):219–20.

32. Tesdahl B, Wilson T, Hoffman H, et al. Epithelial-mesenchymal transition protein expression in basal cell adenomas and basal cell adenocarcinomas. Head Neck Pathol 2016;10:176–81.

33. Cavalcante R, Nonaka C, Santos H, et al. Assessment of *CTNNB1* gene mutations and b-catenin immunoexpression in salivary gland pleomorphic adenomas and adenoid cystic carcinomas. Virchows Arch 2018;472(6):999–1005.

34. Chandrashekar C, Angadi P, Krishnapillai R. B-catenin expression in benign and malignant salivary gland tumors. Int J Surg Pathol 2011;19(4):433–40.

35. Fonseca I, Fonseca R, Martins C, et al. Alteration of b-catenin localization in salivary pleomorphic adenomas is not related to t(3;8)(p21;q12) and is mainly present in non-epithelial cell types. Histopathology 2007;52:239–62.

36. West R, Kong C, Clarke N, et al. MYB expression and translocation in adenoid cystic carcinomas and other salivary gland tumors with clinicopathologic correlation. Am J Surg Pathol 2011;35(1):92–9.

37. Rooney S, Robinson R. Immunohistochemical expression of myb in salivary gland basal cell adenocarcinoma and basal cell adenoma. J Oral Pathol Med 2017;46:798–802.

38. Khurram S, Speight P. Characterisation of DOG-1 expression in salivary gland tumours and comparison with myoepithelial markers. Head Neck Pathol 2019;13:140–8.

39. Andrade E, Teixeira L, Montalli V, et al. Epithelial membrane antigen and DOG1 expression in minor salivary gland tumours. Ann Diagn Pathol 2019;43: 151408.

40. Katabi N, Xu B, Jungbluth AA, et al. PLAG1 immunohistochemistry is a sensitive marker for pleomorphic adenoma: A comparative study with PLAG1 genetic abnormalities. Histopathology 2018;72(2):285–93.

41. Hsieh MS, Lee YH, Chang YL. SOX10-positive salivary gland tumors: a growing list, including mammary analogue secretory carcinoma of the salivary gland, sialoblastoma, low-grade salivary duct carcinoma, basal cell adenoma/adenocarcinoma, and a subgroup of mucoepidermoid carcinoma. Hum Pathol 2016;56:134–42.

42. Liu F, Wang S. Molecular cues for development and regeneration of salivary glands. Histol Histopathol 2014;29(3):305–12.

43. Patel N, Sharpe T, Miletich I. Coordination of epithelial branching and salivary gland lumen formation by Wnt and FGF signals. Dev Biol 2011;358(1):156–67.

44. Prakash S, Swaminathan U, Nagamalini B, et al. Beta-catenin in disease. J Oral Maxillofac Pathol 2016;20(2):289–99.

45. Aberle H, Bauer A, Stappert J, et al. Beta-catenin is a target for the ubiquitin-proteasome pathway. EMBO J 1997;16(13):3797–804.

46. Verhoeft K, Ngan H, Lui V. The cylindromatosis (CYLD) gene and head and neck tumorigenesis. Cancers Head Neck 2016;1:10.

47. Tauriello D, Haegebarth A, Kuper I, et al. Loss of the tumor suppressor CYLD enhances Wnt/beta-catenin signaling through K63-linked ubiquitination of Dvl. Mol Cell 2010;37(5):607–19.

48. Wilson T, Ma D, Tilak A, et al. Next-generation sequencing in salivary gland basal cell adenocarcinoma and basal cell adenoma. Head Neck Pathol 2016;10:494–500.

49. Daa T, Kashima K, Kaku N, et al. Mutations in components of the *wnt* signaling pathway in adenoid cystic carcinoma. Mod Pathol 2004;17(12): 1475–82.

50. Kas K, Voz L, Roijer E, et al. Promoter swapping between the genes for a novel zinc finger protein and beta-catenin in pleiomorphic adenomas with t(3;8)(p21;q12) translocations. Nat Genet 1997; 15(2):170–4.

51. Asahina M, Saito T, Hayashi T, et al. Clinicopatholog-ical effect of PLAG1 fusion genes in pleomorphic adenoma and carcinoma ex pleomorphic adenoma with special emphasis on histological features. Histology 2019;7474(3):514–25.

52. Kazakov DV. Brooke-Spiegler syndrome and pheno-typic variants: an update. Head Neck Pathol 2016; 10(2):125–30.

53. Rito M, Mitani Y, Bell D, et al. Frequent and differen-tial mutations of the CYLD gene in basal cell salivary neoplasms: linkage to tumor development and pro-gression. Mod Pathol 2018;31(7):1064–72.

54. Saida K, Murase T, Ito M, et al. Mutation analysis of the EGFR pathway genes: EGFR, RAS, PIK3CA, BRAF, and Akt1, in salivary gland adenoid cystic carcinoma. Oncotarget 2018;9(24):17043–55.

55. Luk P, Weston J, Yu B, et al. Salivary duct carci-noma: cinicopathologic features, morphologic spec-trum, and somatic mutations. Head Neck 2016; 38(Suppl 1):E1838–47.

Sialadenoma Papilliferum

Min-Shu Hsieh, MD, PhD[a,b], Justin A. Bishop, MD[c],
Julia Yu Fong Chang, DDS, MS, PhD[d,e],*

KEYWORDS

- Sialadenoma papilliferum • Classic • Oncocytic • BRAF V600E mutation • HRAS Q61R mutation

Key points

- Sialadenoma papilliferum (SP) consists of 2 distinct subtypes: (1) classic SP, which is strongly SOX10 positive and genetically analogous to syringocystadenoma papilliferum with consistent BRAF V600E mutations; and (2) oncocytic SP, which is SOX10 negative and is BRAF wild-type.

- SOX10 immunohistochemistry and BRAF analysis (either by immunohistochemistry or molecular testing) may be useful diagnostic adjuncts when confronted with a challenging intraoral salivary gland neoplasm.

- Both the squamous epithelium and ductal epithelium harbor BRAF V600E mutation; thus, both components are neoplastic.

- HRAS Q61R has been shown in 1 SP case.

ABSTRACT

Sialadenoma papilliferum (SP) is a rare, benign salivary gland neoplasm sharing similar histopathologic features and harboring the same genetic alterations, BRAF V600E or HRAS mutations, with syringocystadenoma papilliferum. SP most commonly occurs in the hard palate and in older adults. Clinically, SP is most likely to be diagnosed as a squamous papilloma. Microscopically, SP shows an exophytic papillary epithelial proliferation and a contiguously endophytic ductal proliferation. Two distinct subtypes are identified: classic SP and oncocytic SP. Conservative surgical treatment seems to be adequate with a low recurrence. SOX10 immunohistochemistry and BRAF analysis may be useful in differential diagnosis.

OVERVIEW

Sialadenoma papilliferum (SP) is a rare benign salivary gland neoplasm with the characteristic features of both exophytic papillary proliferation and subjacent ductal proliferation, and therefore it has been categorized as a ductal papilloma. In the ductal papilloma category, both inverted papilloma and intraductal papilloma show intraluminal papillary epithelial proliferation and thus clinically usually appear as a submucosal nodule similar to other salivary gland neoplasms, with some exceptional inverted papillomas showing a craterlike opening at the mucosal surface,[1] which might cause some confusion with SP. Exophytic ductal papilloma, as the nomenclature indicates, shows exophytic ductal epithelial proliferation fused with surface epithelium, and thus clinically it shares similar features with squamous papilloma and SP. However, exophytic ductal papilloma lacks the proliferation of convoluted ductal structures beneath the mucosal epithelium. Therefore, because of the unique histopathologic features of both exophytic and ductal proliferation, SP is readily recognized despite its rare incidence.

SP was first named by Abrams and Finck[2] in 1969 based on the similar histopathologic features to the syringadenoma papilliferum of sweat gland

[a] Department of Pathology, National Taiwan University Hospital, No 7, Chung-Shan South Road, Taipei 100, Taiwan; [b] Graduate Institute of Pathology, National Taiwan University College of Medicine, Taipei, Taiwan; [c] Department of Pathology, University of Texas Southwestern Medical Center, 5323 Harry Hines Boulevard, Dallas, TX 75390, USA; [d] Department of Dentistry, National Taiwan University Hospital, No. 1, Changde Street, Zhongzheng District, Taipei City 100, Taiwan; [e] Department of Dentistry, Graduate Institute of Clinical Dentistry, School of Dentistry, National Taiwan University, Taipei, Taiwan
* Corresponding author.
E-mail address: jyfchang@ntu.edu.tw

Surgical Pathology 14 (2021) 43–51
https://doi.org/10.1016/j.path.2020.09.006
1875-9181/21/© 2020 Elsevier Inc. All rights reserved.

surgpath.theclinics.com

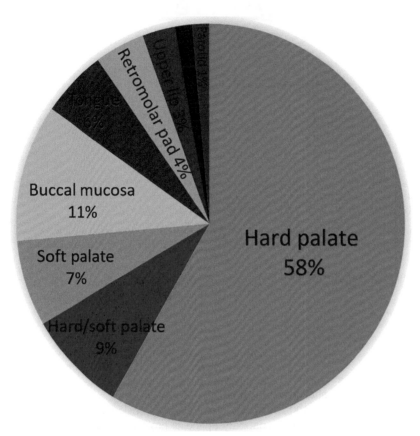

Fig. 1. Anatomic location of SP. (*Data from* Refs.[6–8,15])

origin. Because of their rarity, most SP cases are reported as case reports and in literature reviews. Based on Armed Forces Institute of Pathology data[1] and some large series,[3,4] SP only comprises 0.4% to 1.2% of minor salivary gland tumors. Some large series and extensive literature reviews, including Brannon and colleagues,[5] Fowler and Damm,[6] Hsieh and colleagues,[7] and Nakaguro and colleagues,[8] provide an outline of this rare distinct disease. SP mainly occurs in minor salivary glands and only a few cases are reported in major salivary glands[1,2,5] and other sites, such as bronchus[9] and nasopharynx.[10] There are few case reports[11–14] of malignant transformation of SP; however, because of the presence of some features not consistent with SP, the malignant transformation potential of SP is uncertain. Seventy-two cases from Fowler and Damm,[6] Hsieh and colleagues,[7] Nakaguro and colleagues,[8] and Miyamoto and colleagues[15] were analyzed in this review.

CLINICAL FINDINGS

The most common location for SP is the palate (53 out of 72, 74%), mostly the hard palate (42 out of 72, 58%). The buccal mucosa is the second most common site (8 out of 72, 11%), with few cases involving other locations (**Fig. 1**). SP tends to occur in older adults, and the age range is between 2 and 91 years, with an average age of 60.4 years and peak incidence from 50 to 79 years (**Fig. 2**). SP cases show a slight male predominant (female/male = 1:1.5). However, because of the rarity of SP, some bias might exist. Intraoral SPs are small, ranging from 0.2 to 2.3 cm, with an average size of 0.7 cm. The exceptional parotid SP reported by Abrams and Finck[2] was 7.5 cm in diameter. The most common clinical diagnosis is squamous papilloma,[1,6] with durations ranging from several months to years.[1,6,16]

GROSS FEATURES

Grossly, SP is a well-demarcated papillary or pebbly lesion with sessile or pedunculated base. Both the exophytic papillary projections and endophytic nodular base are less than 1 cm. Some cystic spaces might be seen.[1]

MICROSCOPIC FEATURES

SP shows characteristic histopathologic features of an exophytic proliferation of papillary stratified

Fig. 2. Age distribution of SP. (*Data from* Refs.[6–8,15])

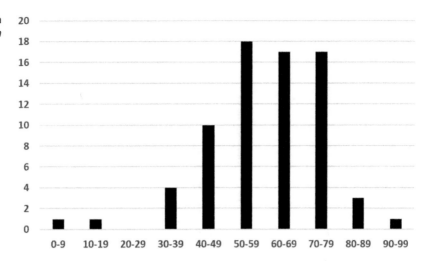

squamous epithelium and a contiguously endophytic salivary ductal proliferation underneath in low-power view (**Fig. 3**A, B). The papillary surface is covered by parakeratinized squamous epithelium and some elongated, branching ductal structures merge with surface squamous epithelium and are revealed as clefts between papillary squamous projections. The ductal proliferation is unencapsulated and classically shows multiple small ducts with irregular luminal contour caused by epithelial folds or papillary structures growing into lumen, and thus reveals fissures or stellatelike luminal spaces (**Fig. 3**C). This ductal epithelium is double layered, with luminal cuboidal to columnar cells and cuboidal to flattened basal cells (**Fig. 3**D). There is usually a mixed lymphoplasmacytic cell infiltrate in the fibrovascular tissues of the papillae and the lamina propria (see **Fig. 3**B, C). Most SPs show superficial ductal proliferation without infiltration into adjacent minor salivary glands (see **Fig. 3**A), but some reveal an infiltrative pattern into the glands (see **Fig. 3**B). Some SPs show 1 or 2 prominently dilated luminal spaces with elongated papillary projections growing inside, which

Fig. 3. Classic type of SP with exophytic papillary surface and underneath ductal proliferation and fissure or stellatelike luminal spaces. (*A*) Classic SP showing a papillary squamous surface and a contiguously endophytic ductal proliferation (original magnification ×40). (*B*) The endophytic ductal proliferation sometimes extends deeply into underlying minor salivary glands (original magnification ×40). (*C*) Ductal epithelium merges with the squamous epithelium (original magnification ×400). (*D*) The ductal cells are composed of columnar to cuboidal cells and arranged in bilayered to multilayered structures (original magnification ×40).

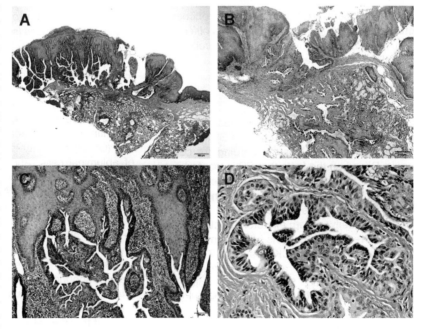

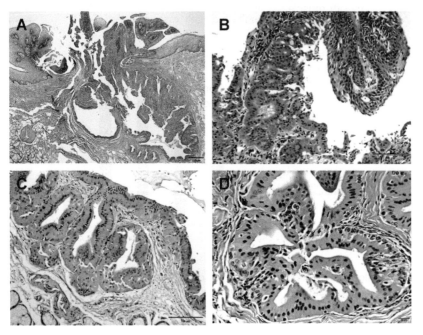

Fig. 4. Oncocytic type of SP with exophytic papillary surface and underneath ductal proliferation. Oncocytic change of the ductal epithelium and less prominent fissure or stellatelike luminal spaces. (*A*) Oncocytic variant of SP has a similar arrangement with both exophytic papillary surface and an endophytic ductal component (original magnification ×40). (*B*) The oncocytic ductal cells merge with overlying stratified squamous epithelium and form papillary structures (original magnification ×40). (*C*) Oncocytic variant of SP shows less prominent fissure or stellatelike spaces (original magnification ×400). (*D*) Oncocytic variant of SP composed of oncocytic cells with round nuclei, abundant eosinophilic cytoplasm, and bland-looking nuclei (original magnification ×40).

slightly resemble the histologic features of intraductal papilloma (**Fig. 4**A). Because of the presence of both exophytic papillary projections and underlying ductal epithelium proliferation, these cases are still SP by definition. Interestingly, these cases frequently show prominent oncocytic changes of the papillary epithelial proliferation (**Fig. 4**B–D). Some mucous goblet cells (see **Fig. 4**B) can also been seen.

IMMUNOHISTOCHEMICAL FINDINGS

Several immunohistochemical studies have been used to identify the cell of origin of SP,[6,17,18] but there is still some debate regarding its cell of origin. Based on the facts that SP is located near the surface epithelium, where the excretory ducts reside, and SP contains both ductal and myoepithelial cells, it has been hypothesized that SP is most likely derived from excretory duct or excretory duct reserve cell origins.[6,17] The immunohistochemical studies for CK13 and CK7 highlight the surface epithelial and proliferative ductal areas, respectively. Some ductal epithelium extending to the surface squamous epithelium of the duct opening can be seen in CK7 immunostain (**Fig. 5**). The basal and spinous cell layers of the squamous epithelium and the basal cell layers of the ductal structures are positive for p63 (**Fig. 6**).

In classic, nononcocytic SP, the p63-positive cells are limited to the basal cell layer of the outer ductal structures (see **Fig. 6**A, C). In oncocytic SP, the p63-positive cells are not only at the outer ductal structures but also at the basal cell layers of the papillary epithelial projections inside the large dilated ductal spaces (see **Fig. 6**B, D). The luminal ductal cells have also shown strong positivity to CK19, S-100,[17] and Epithelial membrane antigen (EMA).[6] Two distinct subsets of the basal or abluminal cells have been identified through different immunophenotypes. One subset shows strong CK14, Smooth muscle actin (SMA), S100, and vimentin positivity. Focal glial fibrillary acidic protein (GFAP) positivity is also seen in this subset of abluminal cells. Another subset shows CK13 and CK14 positivity and is negative for SMA, vimentin, S100, and GFAP.[17] The abluminal cells have also shown p40 immunoreactivity.[6] Some CD1a-positive Langerhans cells distributed inside SPs have also been identified,[17] but their role is unclear.

Notably, the proliferative ductal cells in all classic, nononcocytic SPs are positive for SOX10 (**Fig. 7**A, C), but the ductal cells in oncocytic SPs are negative for SOX10 (**Fig. 7**B, D). These results suggest that the cell of origin for classic, nononcocytic SP is different from that of oncocytic SP. The classic, nononcocytic SP is most likely derived

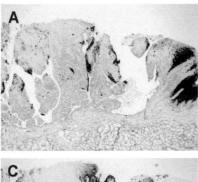
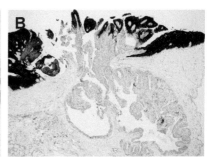
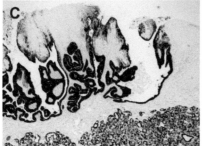
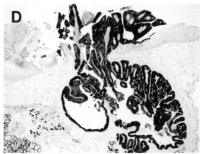

Fig. 5. Immunohistochemical studies for CK13 (*A, B*) and CK7 (*C, D*) on classic and oncocytic type of SP highlight the surface squamous epithelium and ductal epithelium (original magnification ×40).

from intercalated duct or ductal progenitor cells.[19–21] In contrast, oncocytic SP might derive from striated or excretory duct–derived cells based on the SOX10 expression pattern.

MOLECULAR FINDINGS

Recently, *BRAF* V600E mutation was identified in some patients with syringadenoma papilliferum.[22–25] Because SP shares some similar histologic features with syringadenoma papilliferum, the *BRAF* V600E mutation status was recently investigated through *BRAF* V600E mutation–specific immunohistochemical studies and Sanger sequencing by Hsieh and colleagues[7] and Nakaguro and colleagues.[8] Interestingly, *BRAF* VE1 immunohistochemistry was positive in 9 of 9 classic SPs. The staining was cytoplasmic in distribution, and its intensity was weak (1+) in 7 out of 9 patients and moderate (2+) in 2 out of 9 patients (**Fig. 8**A–C). For all 9 classic SPs, *BRAF* VE1 immunoexpression was present in both the ductal and squamous tumor elements, although the intensity of staining was stronger in the ductal component (see **Fig. 8**A). *BRAF* VE1 immunohistochemistry is uniformly negative in all oncocytic SPs (**Fig. 8**D). In cases with sufficient tissue available to be tested for *BRAF* mutation using Sanger sequencing, the *BRAF* c.1799T>A mutation resulting in a p.Val600Glu substitution is confirmed to be present in these classic SPs, whereas the oncocytic SPs are *BRAF* wild-type. In the patients tested by Hsieh and colleagues,[7,20] *HRAS* mutations (codons 12 and 13) tested negative in both

classic-type and oncocytic-type SPs. In the study by Nakaguro and colleagues,[8] showed 7 out of 10 SPs cases were *BRAF* V600E mutated and 1 was *HRAS* Q61R mutated. No differences in histologic features of *BRAF* and/or *HRAS* wild or mutated types were found by Nakaguro and colleagues.[8] A few cases with papillary cystic proliferation but flat surface epithelium, which were categorized as SP-like intraductal papillary tumor (IPT) by Nakaguro and colleagues,[8] have been shown to harbor *BRAF* V600E mutation. One SP-like IPT had both *BRAF* V600E and *HRAS* Q61R mutations.

According to these 2 current molecular studies of SP,[7,8] cases with a classic endophytic component that shows multiple dilated, irregularly branched ductal spaces, intraluminal projections, and fissurelike or stellatelike luminal spaces tend to have *BRAF* V600E mutation. The results might raise the question of whether classic SP and oncocytic SP should be separated because of different morphology, immunophenotype, and genetic alteration.

DIFFERENTIAL DIAGNOSIS

Clinically, SP is easily mistaken for squamous papilloma, verrucous hyperplasia, or exophytic ductal papilloma. Squamous papilloma and verrucous hyperplasia show only squamous epithelial proliferation and thus can be separated from SP easily. Exophytic ductal papilloma has exophytic papillary ductal epithelial proliferation but lacks the subjacent ductal proliferation underneath the

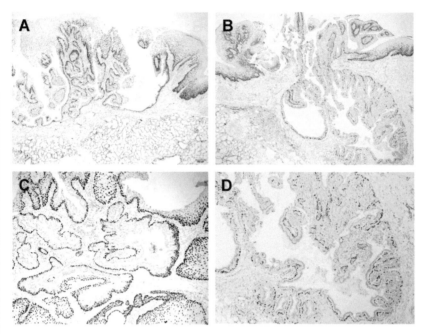

Fig. 6. Immunohistochemical studies for p63 on classic (*A*, *C*) and oncocytic type (*B*, *D*) of SP show the basal cells of the ductal epithelium and squamous epithelium at low and high magnification (original magnification ×40).

epithelium. In immunohistochemical studies, exophytic ductal papilloma is negative for Sox10 and *BRAF* VE1. Intraductal papilloma shows a delicate, branching papillary epithelial proliferation inside a single dilated duct without connection to the surface epithelium. Two intraductal papilloma cases in the study of Nakaguro and colleagues[8] were negative for *BRAF* V600E and *HRAS* Q61R mutations. Inverted papilloma shows endophytic papillary growth occupying most of the luminal space without the exophytic papillary structures and proliferation of small ductal structures seen in SP. Cystadenoma shows a multicystic growth pattern with proliferative, frequently papillary epithelial lining, with the histopathologic findings sometimes overlapping with the inner ductal proliferation component of SP. However, from the lack of exophytic papillary proliferation component of SP, cystadenoma can be easily differentiated from SP. Because of the presence of 3 different kinds

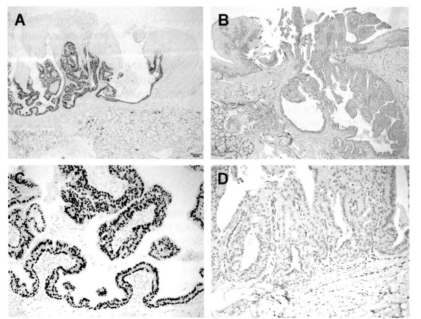

Fig. 7. Immunohistochemical studies for SOX10 on classic (*A*, *C*) and oncocytic type of SP (*B*, *D*) show positive staining for SOX10 in classic SP, but are consistently negative in oncocytic SP at low and high magnification (original magnification ×40).

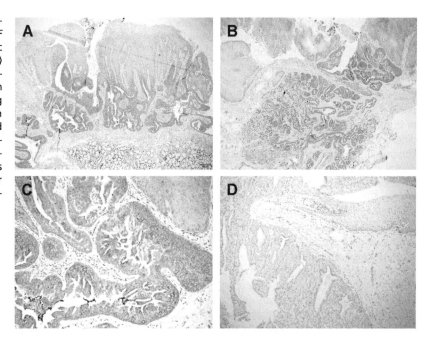

Fig. 8. Immunohistochemical studies for *BRAF* V600E (VE1) in classic (*A–C*) and oncocytic (*D*) SP. (*A–C*) Classic sialadenoma papilliferum showing positive staining for *BRAF* V600E (VE1) in both the glandular and squamous tumor components. (*D*) Oncocytic sialadenoma papilliferum is consistently negative for *BRAF* V600E (VE1) (original magnification ×40).

of cells (squamous, ductal, and mucous cells) in one lesion, unencapsulated border to the architecture, and multiple small ductal proliferations, mucoepidermoid carcinoma is sometimes listed in the differential diagnosis. However, the unique exophytic papillary structures, stellate to fissurelike lumens of the ductal proliferations, and distinct distribution of different cell types in SP readily helps to differentiate it from mucoepidermoid carcinoma.

DIAGNOSIS

- SP shows characteristic histopathologic features of an exophytic proliferation of papillary stratified squamous epithelium and a contiguously endophytic salivary ductal proliferation underneath.
- Immunohistochemically, the proliferative ductal cells in all classic, nononcocytic SPs are positive for SOX10, but the ductal cells in oncocytic SPs are negative for SOX10.
- Genetically, around 70% of SPs show *BRAF* V600E mutation. The classic SPs show 100% *BRAF* V600E mutation, in contrast with wild-type *BRAF* in oncocytic SPs.

PROGNOSIS

Most SPs have a nonaggressive biological behavior and are treated by conservative surgical excision. Although nearly half of the cases lack follow-up information, the rare publications in the literature might indicate no recurrence in most cases. Available follow-up data from a literature review showed a recurrence rate of 7.4% with follow-up periods of 2 to 96 months.[6] A few case reports mentioned possible malignant transformation in SP[11–14,26]; however, the evidence showing malignancy derived from preexisting SP is insufficient.

SUMMARY

SP is a rare, benign salivary gland neoplasm not only sharing similar histopathologic features but also harboring the same genetic alterations (*BRAF* V600E or *HRAS* mutations) with syringocystadenoma papilliferum, an uncommon benign tumor of sweat gland origin. SP most commonly occurs in the palate, especially the hard palate, and most frequently occurs in older adults, with a peak age range of 50 to 79 years. Clinically, SP is most likely to be diagnosed as squamous papilloma. Microscopically, SP shows an exophytic proliferation of papillary stratified squamous epithelium and a contiguously endophytic ductal proliferation underneath. The endophytic component typically shows multiple dilated, irregularly branched ductal spaces lined by bilayered to multilayered epithelial cells with intraluminal projections, giving the luminal spaces a fissurelike or stellatelike appearance. Some oncocytic SPs show identical structures to classic SP, but the ductal components are entirely lined by oncocytic cells and do not have foci of conventional-appearing ductal epithelium. Classic SP and onco-cytic SP show similar patterns of immunostains for CK13, CK7, and p63. CK13 and CK7 highlight the surface squamous epithelial and proliferative ductal areas, respectively, whereas p63 is diffusely positive in the squamous tumor epithelium and positive in the basal layer of the ductal epithelium. In contrast, classic SP and oncocytic SP show different SOX10 expression patterns. Classic SP shows diffuse and strong SOX10 positivity in the ductal component but is completely negative in all oncocytic SPs. Around 70% of SPs, mainly classic SP, are *BRAF* V600E mutated, and 1 SP was *HRAS* Q61R mutated. Oncocytic SPs are *BRAF* wild-type. Conservative surgical treatment seems to be adequate, with a recurrence rate of 7.4% documented.

In summary, recent studies have used histolog-ic, immunophenotypic, and molecular analysis to shed light on this rare salivary gland tumor. The SP group consists of 2 distinct subtypes: (1) classic SP, which is strongly SOX10 positive and genetically analogous to syringocystadenoma papilliferum with consistent *BRAF* V600E muta-tions; and (2) oncocytic SP, which is SOX10 nega-tive and is *BRAF* wild-type. These findings further refine salivary gland tumor classification and sug-gest that SOX10 immunohistochemistry and *BRAF* analysis (either by immunohistochemistry or molecular testing) may be useful diagnostic ad-juncts when confronted with a challenging intrao-ral salivary gland neoplasm.

CLINICS CARE POINTS

- SP is a rare, benign salivary gland neoplasm most frequently occurring in the hard palate of older adults.

- Conservative surgical removal seems to be adequate, with a low recurrence.

- SOX10 immunohistochemistry and BRAF analysis may be useful in differential diag-nosis.

ACKNOWLEDGEMENTS

This work was supported by the Ministry of Sci-ence and Technology, ROC [MOST 108-2314-B-002-039-]; National Taiwan University Hospital grant [108-N4355]; and the National Health Research Institutes [NHRI-EX108-10612EC].

DISCLOSURE

The authors have nothing to disclose.

REFERENCES

1. Ellis GL, Auclair PL. Tumors of the salivary glands. AFIP atlas of tumor pathology, 4th series, fascicle 9. Silver Spring MD: ARP Press; 2008. p. 148–51.
2. Abrams AM, Finck FM. Sialadenoma papilliferum. A previously unreported salivary gland tumor. Cancer 1969;24(5):1057–63.
3. Regezi JA, Lloyd RV, Zarbo RJ, et al. Minor salivary gland tumors. A histologic and immunohistochem-ical study. Cancer 1985;55:108–15.
4. Waldron CA, el-Mofty SK, Gnepp DR. Tumors of the intraoral minor salivary glands: a demographic and histologic study of 426 cases. Oral Surg Oral Med Oral Pathol 1988;66(3):323–33.
5. Brannon RB, Sciubba JJ, Giulani M. Ductal papil-lomas of salivary gland origin: A report of 19 cases and a review of the literature. Oral Surg Oral Med Oral Pathol Oral Radiol Endod 2001;92(1):68–77.
6. Fowler CB, Damm DD. Sialadenoma Papilliferum: Analysis of Seven New Cases and Review of the Literature. Head Neck Pathol 2018;12(2):193–201.
7. Hsieh M-S, Bishop JA, Wang Y-P, et al. Salivary Siala-denoma Papilliferum Consists of Two Morphologically, Immunophenotypically, and Genetically Distinct Sub-types. Head Neck Pathol 2019;14(2):489.
8. Nakaguro M, Urano M, Ogawa I, et al. Histopatho-logical evaluation of minor salivary gland papillary–cystic tumours: focus on genetic alterations in siala-denoma papilliferum and intraductal papillary mucinous neoplasm. Histopathology 2020;76(3): 411–22.
9. Bobos M, Hytiroglou P, Karkavelas G, et al. Sialade-noma papilliferum of bronchus. Virchows Arch 2003; 443(5):695–9.
10. Hamilton J, Osborne RF, Smith LM. Sialadenoma papilliferum involving the nasopharynx. Ear Nose Throat J 2005;84(8):474–5.
11. Solomon MP, Rosen Y, Alfonso A. Intraoral papillary squamous cell tumor of the soft palate with features of sialadenoma papilliferum-? malignant sialade-noma papilliferum. Cancer 1978;42(4):1859–69.
12. Shimoda M, Kameyama K, Morinaga S, et al. Malig-nant transformation of sialadenoma papilliferum of the palate: a case report. Virchows Arch 2004; 445(6):641–6.
13. Ponniah I. A rare case of sialadenoma papilliferum with epithelial dysplasia and carcinoma in situ. Oral Surg Oral Med Oral Pathol Oral Radiol Endod 2007;104(2):e27–9.
14. Liu W, Gnepp DR, de Vries E, et al. Mucoepidermoid carcinoma arising in a background of sialadenoma papilliferum: a case report. Head Neck Pathol 2009;3(1):59–62.
15. Miyamoto S, Ogawa T, Chikazu D. Sialadenoma papilliferum in the buccal mucosa detected on (18)

F-fluorodeoxyglucose-positron emission tomography. Br J Oral Maxillofac Surg 2017;55(7):727–9.

16. Mahajan D, Khurana N, Setia N. Sialadenoma papilliferum in a young patient: a case report and review of the literature. Oral Surg Oral Med Oral Pathol Oral Radiol Endod 2007;103(3):e51–4.

17. Maiorano E, Favia G, Ricco R. Sialadenoma papilliferum: an immunohistochemical study of five cases. J Oral Pathol Med 1996;25:336–42.

18. Ubaidat MA, Robinson RA, Belding PJ, et al. Sialadenoma papilliferum of the hard palate: report of 2 cases and immunohistochemical evaluation. Arch Pathol Lab Med 2001;125(12):1595–7.

19. Athwal HK, Murphy G, Tibbs E, et al. Sox10 Regulates Plasticity of Epithelial Progenitors toward Secretory Units of Exocrine Glands. Stem Cell Reports 2019;12:366–80.

20. Hsieh MS, Lee YH, Chang YL. SOX10-positive salivary gland tumors: a growing list, including mammary analogue secretory carcinoma of the salivary gland, sialoblastoma, low-grade salivary duct carcinoma, basal cell adenoma/adenocarcinoma, and a subgroup of mucoepidermoid carcinoma. Hum Pathol 2016;56:134–42.

21. Ohtomo R, Mori T, Shibata S, et al. SOX10 is a novel marker of acinus and intercalated duct differentiation in salivary gland tumors: a clue to the histogenesis for tumor diagnosis. Mod Pathol 2013;26(8):1041–50.

22. Konstantinova AM, Kyrpychova L, Nemcova J, et al. Syringocystadenoma Papilliferum of the Anogenital Area and Buttocks: A Report of 16 Cases, Including Human Papillomavirus Analysis and HRAS and BRAF V600 Mutation Studies. Am J Dermatopathol 2018. https://doi.org/10.1097/dad.0000000000001285.

23. Levinsohn JL, Sugarman JL, Bilguvar K, et al, The Yale Center For Mendelian Genomics. Somatic V600E BRAF Mutation in Linear and Sporadic Syringocystadenoma Papilliferum. J Invest Dermatol 2015;135:2536–8.

24. Shen AS, Peterhof E, Kind P, et al. Activating mutations in the RAS/mitogen-activated protein kinase signaling pathway in sporadic trichoblastoma and syringocystadenoma papilliferum. Hum Pathol 2015;46(2):272–6.

25. Watanabe Y, Shido K, Niihori T, et al. Somatic BRAF c.1799T>A p.V600E Mosaicism syndrome characterized by a linear syringocystadenoma papilliferum, anaplastic astrocytoma, and ocular abnormalities. Am J Med Genet A 2016;170A(1):189–94.

26. Ide F, Kikuchi K, Kusama K, et al. Sialadenoma papilliferum with potentially malignant features. J Clin Pathol 2010;63(4):362–4.

Papillary Neoplasms of the Salivary Duct System
A Review

Abbas Agaimy, MD

KEYWORDS

- Salivary glands • IPMN • Intraductal papilloma • Cystadenoma • Mucinous • Papillary
- *AKT1* mutations • Intraductal papillary mucinous neoplasm

Key points

- A papillary growth pattern can be encountered in a variety of reactive, benign, low-grade, and high-grade malignant salivary gland lesions.

- Some of these lesions likely represent a biological continuum.

- Besides phenotyping, genetic profiling is emerging as a reproducible discriminator for their diagnostic work-up.

- The historical descriptive term papillary adenocarcinomas refers to a histologic pattern and not an entity, and hence should be abandoned.

- Lack of cytologic atypia in biologically malignant neoplasms and presence of solid-papillary patterns represent pitfalls in correctly identifying these entities.

ABSTRACT

Papillary lesions of the salivary duct systems are uncommon. They encompass a heterogeneous group of benign, intermediate, and potentially aggressive neoplasms. With a few exceptions, historical descriptive terms such as papillary adenocarcinoma, papillary cystadenocarcinoma, and papillary adenoma are being replaced by defined entities, at same time acknowledging the papillary features as a histologic pattern. The evolving genetic landscape of these lesions increasingly permits their reproducible categorization. This article discusses those papillary proliferations encountered in the salivary glands with a focus on intraductal papillary mucinous neoplasms and cystadenomas. Intraductal carcinomas and sialadenoma papilliferum are addressed in separate articles in this issue.

OVERVIEW

The term "papillary" has historically been used loosely to refer to many salivary gland neoplasms characterized by a prominent papillary growth pattern but that have otherwise little in common. This usage resulted in frequent use of merely descriptive terms to refer to diagnostic entities such as papillary cystadenoma, papillary adenocarcinoma, papillary cystadenocarcinoma, adenopapillary carcinoma, ductal papilloma, and other related terminologies. Although these descriptive terms have been used in the sense of tentative entities, well-reproducible diagnostic criteria have generally been lacking. In addition, the defining genetic background of these putative entities until recently remained obscure. Moreover, frequent occurrence of papillary growth pattern in diverse salivary gland entities, albeit to a variable extent, has limited the reproducibility and questioned the

Institute of Pathology, University Hospital, Erlangen, Friedrich-Alexander-University Erlangen-Nürnberg (FAU), Krankenhausstrasse 8-10, 91054 Erlangen, Germany
E-mail address: abbas.agaimy@uk-erlangen.de

surgpath.theclinics.com

Surgical Pathology 14 (2021) 53–65
https://doi.org/10.1016/j.path.2020.09.007
1875-9181/21/© 2020 Elsevier Inc. All rights reserved.

usefulness of these terms as diagnoses. The only exceptions are papillary cystadenoma and ductal papilloma, which survived as diagnostic terms to date.

With the rapidly advancing pathology and molecular biology of salivary gland neoplasms, several entities became well established on reproducible morphologic/phenotypic and, in particular, genotypic basis. This development has resulted in a dynamic refinement of diagnostic categories, recognition and separation of uncommon papillary variants of well-known entities (eg, secretory carcinoma), and establishment of new entities.

At present, a papillary growth pattern is recognized in 2 major groups of salivary gland neoplasms: (1) lesions located within and limited to the duct system (intraductal papillary neoplasms); and (2) invasive salivary gland carcinomas with variable, occasionally prominent, papillary growth pattern (**Table 1**). This article is devoted to those noninvasive papillary lesions.

INTRADUCTAL/INTRACYSTIC PROLIFERATIONS OF THE SALIVARY GLAND DUCT SYSTEM

Papillary and papillary-cystic proliferations of the salivary gland duct system are uncommon. Their rarity precluded establishment of reproducible diagnostic criteria and resulted in the use of ill-defined terms in the old literature, making comparison among different studies difficult or even impossible. For example, cystic lesions with papillary features and oncocytic lining might have been classified as papillary cystadenomas by some investigators, whereas they likely have been lumped into the spectrum of lymphocyte-poor Warthin tumors by others. Likewise, intraductal papillary mucinous neoplasms (IPMNs) have been reported under different names, making their retrieval from the literature difficult. From a cytologic viewpoint, the neoplastic cells in these intraductal proliferations may recapitulate any of the normal ductal cell types or they may adopt a metaplastic cell type not frequently, or not usually, present in the duct system. Lesions may therefore show columnar cells, mucinous cells, epidermoid cells, oncocytic cells, small intermediatelike or intercalated-type cells, or variable combinations thereof. In the current World Health Organization (WHO) classification of salivary gland neoplasms, 3 major subtypes of papillary or papillary-cystic lesions are recognized:

1. Cystadenomas
2. Sialadenoma papilliferum

Table 1
Salivary gland neoplasms with definitional (1–5) or occasional (6–10) papillary growth patterns

No	Tumor Type	Genotype (%)	Biology/Behavior
1	Papillary cystadenoma	No data	Benign
2	Sialadenoma papilliferum, classic	BRAF V600E (100)	Benign
3	Intraductal papilloma	No data	Benign
4	IPMN, noninvasive	AKT1 p.Glu17Lys; E17K (92) HRAS mutation (8)	Benign[a]
5	IPMN, invasive	No data	No data
6	Intraductal carcinoma, intercalated duct type, noninvasive	RET fusions; eg, NCOA4, TRIM27 (58)	Low grade
7	Intraductal carcinoma, intercalated duct type, invasive	RET fusions; eg, NCOA4, TRIM27, (58)	Low grade
8	Papillary secretory carcinoma	ETV6-NTRK, ETV6-RET fusions, others (100)	Low to higher grade[b]
9	Polymorphous adenocarcinoma	PRKD1, PRKD2, PRKD3	Low grade
10	Papillary adenocarcinoma NOS	No data	Variable grades

Abbreviations: IPMN, intraductal papillary mucinous neoplasm; NOS, not otherwise specified.
[a] No sufficient long-term follow-up da.
[b] Based on whether with or without high-grade transformation.

3. Ductal papillomas (including an inverted and an intraductal variant)[1–3]

These lesions, their pertinent differential diagnoses, and recent advances in their molecular pathogenesis are discussed in detail in this article. Intraductal carcinoma and sialadenoma papilliferum as genuine components in the differential diagnostic spectrum of these intraductal papillary lesions are addressed separately in this issue and are only briefly mentioned in the differential diagnosis as necessary.

CYSTADENOMAS

Cystadenomas of salivary glands are uncommon. They represent from 1% to 4% of all salivary gland neoplasms. However, the plethora of names used in the literature (papillary cystadenoma, monomorphic adenoma, cystic duct adenoma, Warthin tumor without lymphoid stroma, intraductal papillary hyperplasia, oncocytic cystadenoma, duct ectasia, and others) precludes any reliable or conclusive assessment of their true incidence.[1,4] Women are more frequently affected than men. The mean age is in the fifth to seventh decade of life. Most papillary cystadenomas originate in the major salivary glands (45% in the parotid gland).[1,4] In contrast, lesions affecting the minor salivary glands are exceptionally rare. In 2015, Tjioe and colleagues[4] reported 11 minor salivary gland cases and found 19 cases reported in the English literature between 1958 and 2014, highlighting the rarity of papillary cystadenoma in the minor salivary glands. The lip and the buccal mucosa are the main 2 sites affected among minor salivary gland lesions. In the minor salivary glands, cystadenomas present clinically as slowly growing painless nodules or masses, usually covered by a smooth mucosal surface, frequently mimicking a mucocele. In the major salivary glands, they present as swellings and, except for variable cystic features, are clinically not distinguishable from other salivary gland adenomas.[1,4]

Based on the cytologic and architectural characteristics, cystadenomas are divided into unicystic and multicystic, papillary, oncocytic, and mucinous variants.

Papillary Cystadenoma

On histology, papillary cystadenoma shows a well-circumscribed, noninvasive, predominantly multicystic growth of variably sized cystic spaces lined by epithelial cells that vary greatly in their differentiation and papillary configuration (Box 1, Fig. 1A–C). At the periphery of the lesion, entrapment of native salivary acini and/or ducts is common.[3,4] Up to 20% of cases are unicystic. The lining epithelium is frequently an admixture of columnar, cuboidal, and oncocytic cells, present in variable combinations (Fig. 1D–F). Squamous, apocrine, and ciliated cells may be present but are uncommon (Fig. 1G–I).[5] Although predominance of oncocytic cells is frequent, hence closely mimicking lymphocyte-poor Warthin tumors, mucinous and squamous cells are only rarely the predominant cell type. Cystadenomas lack cytologic atypia, mitotic activity, and invasive growth. Although the presence of simple papillary projections and a few multiple papillae is a common feature in cystadenomas, the presence of prominent complex papillary tufting should alert pathologists to the possibility of intercalated-type intraductal carcinoma and other entities. Immunohistochemistry is usually not necessary for diagnosis but may be of help to exclude macrocystic secretory carcinoma[6] and, in particular, intercalated-type intraductal carcinoma.[7] The lining cells frequently show a simple luminal phenotype with expression of CK8/18, but, in contrast with intraductal carcinoma, protein S100 and SOX10 are either absent or only focally expressed.[8,9]

Mucinous Cystadenoma

Mucinous cystadenoma has not been established as a distinctive entity but is considered a histologic variant of papillary cystadenoma. It is basically identical to papillary cystadenoma but has a predominance of mucinous columnar cells lining the cysts (Fig. 2A–F). There are no atypia or complex papillary projections.[8,10] The lumens are filled with thick mucoid secretion. The epithelial lining is supported by a basal cell layer.

TREATMENT AND PROGNOSIS

Papillary cystadenoma is cured by simple excision and recurrence is rare. Anecdotal cases of invasive carcinoma originating from a background cystadenoma have been reported.[11,12] One lesion with features of so-called cystadenocarcinoma originating from cystadenoma is shown in Fig. 3.

| Box 1 |
Main features of cystadenomas
Unicystic or multicystic
Well circumscribed, noninfiltrative
Diversity of lining cells
No complex papillae
Basally oriented p63-positive cells

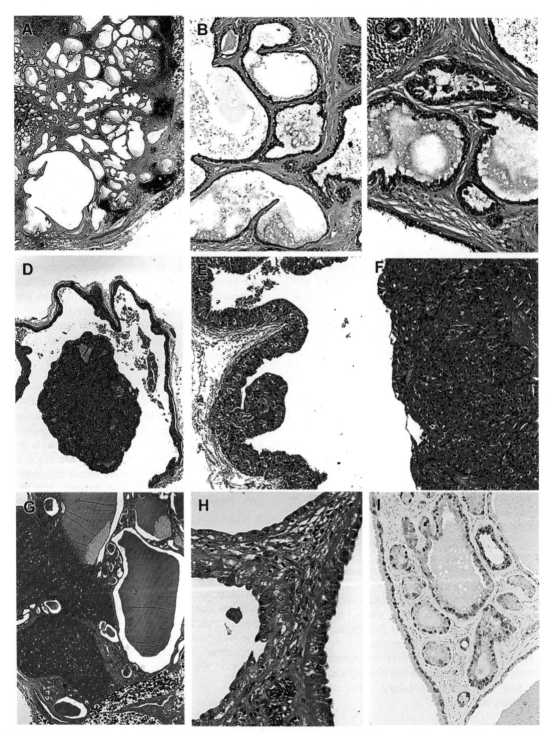

Fig. 1. A cystadenoma showing the characteristic well-circumscribed multicystic growth [hematoxylin-eosin, original magnification ×100] (A), [hematoxylin-eosin, original magnification ×200] (B) (*A*, *B*). The cysts are lined by bland cuboidal bilayered epithelium (*C*; note entrapped normal duct at upper left [hematoxylin-eosin, original magnification ×400]). Unicystic oncocytic papillary cystadenoma closely mimics salivary duct cyst but shows a prominent luminal solid-papillary component [hematoxylin-eosin, original magnification ×100] (*D*). The cyst lumen is lined by a few layers of oncocytic epithelium with papillary infoldings and a few metaplastic mucinous cells, and is bordered by continuous layer of small basal cells [hematoxylin-eosin, original magnification ×200] (*E*). Higher magnification of the solid-papillary component [hematoxylin-eosin, original magnification ×400] (*F*). This example of multicystic cystadenoma [hematoxylin-eosin, original magnification ×100] (*G*) is lined predominantly by apocrine type eosinophilic cells [hematoxylin-eosin, original magnification ×400] (*H*) bordered by a continuous basal layer highlighted by S100 immunostaining (*I*).

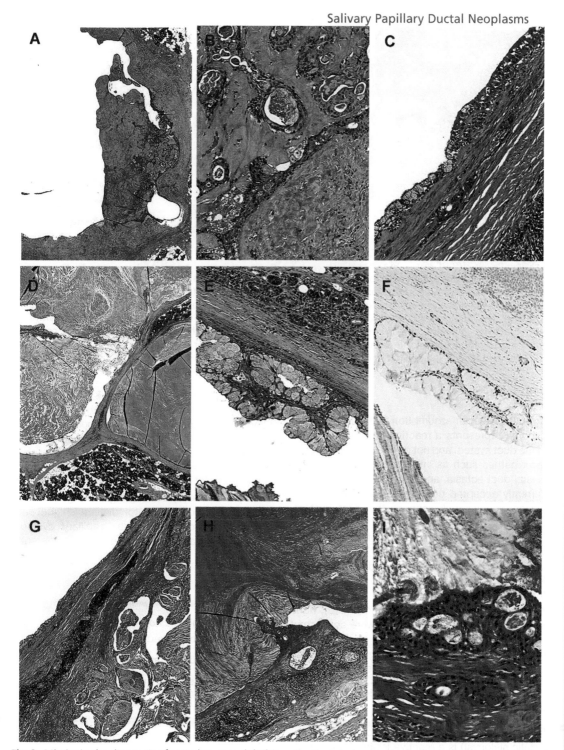

Fig. 2. Mimics in the diagnosis of cystadenomas. (*A*) This unicystic cystadenoma had a focal papillary intraluminal component with prominent regressive changes, sclerosis, and squamous reaction/metaplasia entrapping a few mucous cells mimicking low-grade mucoepidermoid carcinoma (hematoxylin-eosin, original magnification ×50). (*B*) The cystic wall is lined by combination of oncocytic (*upper right*) and mucous cells (*C; lower left*) [hematoxylin-eosin, original magnification ×100] (*B*), [hematoxylin-eosin, original magnification ×100] (*C*). (*D*) This multicystic purely mucinous cystadenoma is hardly ever distinguishable from mucous cell–rich mucoepidermoid carcinoma (hematoxylin-eosin, original magnification ×50). The mucous cells showed flat papillary infoldings [hematoxylin-eosin, original magnification ×200] (*E*) and are bordered by a strictly basal continuous layer of p63-positive cells (*F*). (*G–I*) This predominantly cystic low-grade mucoepidermoid carcinoma is very similar to the cystadenoma in (*C–F*) [hematoxylin-eosin, original magnification ×50] (*G*). The few focal papillae [hematoxylin-eosin, original magnification ×50] (*H*) are composed of small intermediate cells and a few mucous cells [hematoxylin-eosin, original magnification ×200] (*I*). All these examples have been verified by *MAML2* gene fusion testing.

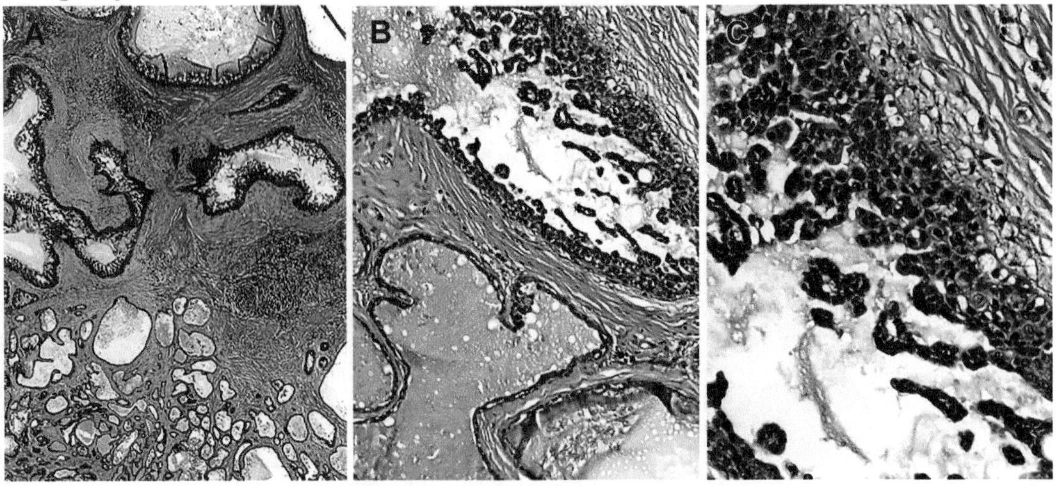

Fig. 3. Example of malignant transformation of cystadenoma. (*A, B*) This unusual example (from deep parotid gland lobe) shows transition from conventional multicystic cystadenoma (*lower field*) to an atypical component (*upper field*) [hematoxylin-eosin, original magnification ×100] (*A*), [hematoxylin-eosin, original magnification ×200] (*B*). The latter reveals complex hierarchical papillary tufts lined by monomorphic atypical cells with brisk mitotic activity [hematoxylin-eosin, original magnification ×400] (*C*). The immunophenotype was consistent with intraductal carcinoma of intercalated duct type (strongly positive for CK7, S100, SOX10, and mammaglobin with retained basal cell layer; data not shown).

GENETIC FEATURES

Against the earlier assumption that salivary cystadenoma represents a reactive cystic hyperplasia of the duct system and not a true neoplasm (hence older names such as intraductal papillary hyperplasia, duct ectasia, and salivary duct cysts), it is currently accepted that cystadenomas represent benign neoplastic lesions of the duct system, albeit of uncertain molecular pathogenesis.[1] To date, no data exist on the genetic findings in conventional papillary cystadenomas. Three cystadenomas (2 oncocytic) were analyzed in the study by Nakaguro and colleagues,[13] who used an assay for detection of mutations in 6 genes (*BRAF, AKT1, PIK3CA, HRAS, KRAS,* and *GNAS*); none showed a mutation. A few cases were concurrent with Warthin tumor, which, based on their shared oncocytic phenotype, might suggest a common pathogenesis, but this remains speculative.[14]

DIFFERENTIAL DIAGNOSIS

Intraoral salivary duct cyst (ductal ectasia or ectatic sialocyst) is a reactive lesion, likely resulting from luminal obstruction (**Box 2**). The buccal region, the lower lip, the mandibular vestibule, and the mouth floor are the main sites involved.[15] Intraoral salivary duct cysts show a variety of epithelial linings, including oncocytic, mucinous, and squamous. Papillary infoldings or undulations and oncocytic metaplasia mimicking papillary oncocytic cystadenoma are observed in 22% of cases.[15]

A few immunohistochemical studies aimed to identify distinguishing features between mucoepidermoid carcinoma and cystadenoma. A strictly basal p63 pattern is observed in cystadenomas and is in contrast with the disordered nonorganoid or nonbasal reactivity of p63 in mucoepidermoid carcinoma.[16,17] Analysis of the apomucin profiles was performed by some groups trying to find out differential expression to distinguish between mucoepidermoid carcinoma, papillary cystadenoma, and salivary duct cyst.[17] No differential

---

Box 2
Main differential diagnoses of cystadenomas

Oncocytic and eosinophilic cystadenomas:
- Cystic oncocytic mucoepidermoid carcinoma
- Cystic oncocytic myoepithelioma
- Oncocytic salivary duct cyst with undulations
- Oncocytic intercalated duct-type intraductal carcinoma
- Macrocystic secretory carcinoma
- Low-grade apocrine intraductal carcinoma
- Intraductal papillomas/IPMN

Mucinous cystadenomas:
- Mucocele or predominantly mucinous salivary duct cyst
- Unicystic or multicystic mucoepidermoid carcinoma

expression was found between the 3 entities regarding positive expression of MUC1, MUC2, MUC4, and MUC7. However, negativity with MUC1 and MUC4 was found to be in favor of a benign diagnosis (papillary cystadenoma or salivary duct cyst).

The most striking features that permit distinction of papillary cystadenoma from its mimics is the prominent multicystic growth with more lumens than epithelial cells at low power. The presence of prominent complex or arborizing papillae and tufting should alert pathologists to the possibility of intercalated-type intraductal carcinoma (**Fig.** 4A–C) or IPMN (discussed later). Likewise,

macrocystic secretory carcinoma may on occasion be hardly distinguishable from papillary cystadenomas (**Fig.** 4D–F). There are insufficient data on the value of S100 and mammaglobin expression as discriminators between papillary cystadenoma and secretory carcinoma and intercalated-type intraductal carcinoma. However, the monomorphic small to medium-sized intercalated-type cells of intraductal carcinoma and the prominent pseudoinfiltrative noncircumscribed growth filling and dilating the ducts with frequent sievelike appearance is characteristic of intraductal carcinoma and is absent in papillary cystadenoma.[7] Intraductal carcinoma and secretory carcinoma

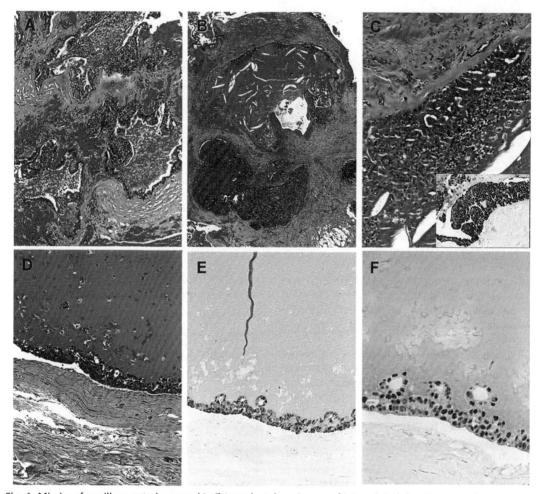

Fig. 4. Mimics of papillary cystadenoma. (*A–C*) Intraductal carcinoma of intercalated duct type may show a prominent cystic-papillary pattern indistinguishable from papillary cystadenoma (some archival cases have been originally diagnosed as such). Lobular pattern and presence of solid or sievelike component should always suggest intraductal carcinoma. (*C, inset*) Diffuse mammaglobin reactivity [hematoxylin-eosin, original magnification ×100] (*A*), [hematoxylin-eosin, original magnification ×100] (*B*), [hematoxylin-eosin, original magnification ×200] (*C*). This recurrent macrocystic secretory carcinoma (carrying the canonical *ETV6-NTRK3* fusion) was very suggestive of unicystic papillary cystadenoma [hematoxylin-eosin, original magnification ×100] (*D*). The neoplastic cells homogeneously expressed S100 (*E*) and pan-TRK antibody, the latter with nuclear pattern (*F*).

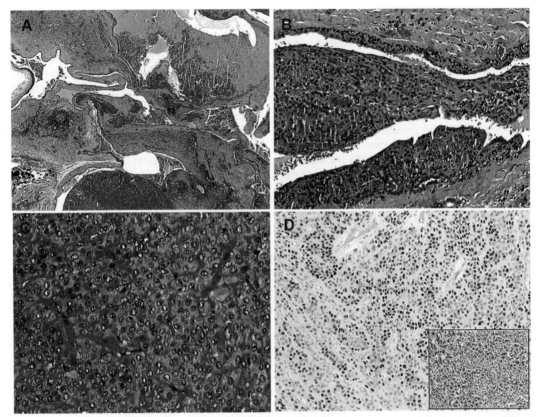

Fig. 5. (*A*) This example of oncocytoid myoepithelioma of the parotid gland showed a preeminently multicystic growth very similar to cystadenoma and contained a focal solid component (*lower field*) [hematoxylin-eosin, original magnification ×50]. (*B*) In some areas, apically oriented oncocytic cells are surrounded by multiple layers of small basaloid cells forming flat papillary structures [hematoxylin-eosin, original magnification ×100]. (*C*) Higher magnification of the solid component [hematoxylin-eosin, original magnification ×200]. (*D*) Homogeneous expression of p63 (*main image*) and S100 (*inset*) in the solid component.

are uniformly immunoreactive with S100 and mammaglobin.[7,18] At the molecular level, they harbor frequent *NCOA4-RET* or *TRIM27-RET* gene fusions (intraductal carcinoma is discussed elsewhere in this issue).[7,19]

A major consideration in mucinous cystadenomas is the macrocystic variant of mucoepidermoid carcinoma (**Fig. 2**G–I). Distinction in some cases is arbitrary, because some unicystic or multicystic mucoepidermoid carcinomas contain no more than minimal solid foci attached to the cyst lining or floating within the luminal secretion. Recognition of such foci should alert pathologists to the possibility of multicystic mucoepidermoid carcinoma and justify molecular testing for an *MAML2* gene fusion. Rare mucoepidermoid carcinomas were thought to have their origin within salivary duct cysts.[20] Furthermore, multicystic mucoepidermoid carcinoma may have luminal papillary projections that, in turn, may closely mimic papillary or mucinous cystadenoma. A variety of other benign and malignant salivary neoplasms occasionally

show a prominent papillary-cystic configuration hardly distinguishable from papillary cystadenoma (**Fig. 5**).

INTRADUCTAL PAPILLOMA AND INTRADUCTAL PAPILLARY MUCINOUS NEOPLASMS

Intraductal Papilloma

The term intraductal papilloma has been used loosely to refer to neoplasms characterized by prominent papillary growth within a salivary duct and lacking diagnostic criteria of other entities in the absence of features of malignancy.[3] In the past, ductal papillomas have been subdivided into intraductal papillomas and inverted ductal papillomas.[3]

The incidence of ductal papillomas remains poorly characterized, but they are exceedingly rare, with no more than 50 cases reported to date.[21,22] Although many have likely been underdiagnosed as cystadenomas, others are possibly overdiagnosed. Intraductal papillomas represented 0.3% of all salivary epithelial neoplasms and 0.5% of benign tumors in the Armed Forced Institute of Pathology salivary gland database.[23] Most originate in the terminal excretory duct portions of the intraoral minor salivary glands, with the lips, floor of mouth, buccal mucosa, palate, and tongue as main sites. The major salivary glands are only rarely involved.[21,22]

Although inverted ductal papillomas are easily recognized from their prominent squamous differentiation and characteristic endophytic growth close to the surface,[3] intraductal papillomas have been poorly defined. An epidermoid component is often mentioned in intraductal papillomas, but this seems rare or unusual.

Histologic Features

Looking at the literature, lesions that were microscopic or predominantly small (up to 5 mm) and composed of a few papillary projections within a slightly dilated duct have been reported as intraductal papilloma. In contrast, tumors composed of highly aggregated complex papillary tufts distending and dilating the involved duct segment were similarly named intraductal papilloma (**Fig. 6**). These observations suggest the existence of a spectrum of intraductal papillary proliferations ranging from microscopic foci to well-circumscribed larger cellular and complex proliferating papillary lesions involving continuously or discontinuously larger duct segments or the whole duct system. This phenomenon is highly reminiscent of the intraductal proliferations of the breast and the pancreatobiliary system. The author therefore prefers to separate these lesions from classic intraductal papillomas and they are discussed hereafter as IPMN (**Table 2**).

Genetic Findings

There are currently no data on the genetic features of intraductal papillomas after separation of the IPMN type. Only 2 cases of papilloma were included in the genetic study by Nakaguro and colleagues,[13] who used an assay for detection of mutations in 6 genes (BRAF, AKT1, PIK3CA, HRAS, KRAS, and GNAS); none showed a mutation.

INTRADUCTAL PAPILLARY MUCINOUS NEOPLASMS OF THE SALIVARY GLANDS

Recently, our group described 3 cases of low-grade salivary gland neoplasms in the histologic spectrum of intraductal papillomas, but showed in addition increasing cytologic and architectural atypia of variable extent and degree with easily identifiable mitoses and variable, striking similarity to pancreatobiliary IPMN and occasionally mimicry of low-grade ductal carcinoma in situ of the breast.[24] The spectrum of growth pattern and the degree of atypia in these intraductal papillary growths point to a lesion with a potential for malignant transformation. The term IPMN has been proposed to reflect and accommodate variations on the spectrum of these potentially malignant intraductal papillary proliferations in analogy to their pancreatobiliary counterparts.[25]

The incidence of salivary IPMN is unknown because it is difficult to retrieve cases of IPMN with or without malignant transformation from the older literature because of the plethora of confusing terms used by different investigators. It seems that most lesions might have been lumped into the category of intraductal papillomas.[21] In addition, it seems that at least some cases hide behind terms such as mucinous cystadenocarcinoma, mucus cell adenocarcinoma, mucus-producing adenopapillary carcinoma, high-grade papillary cystadenocarcinoma, and papillary cystadenoma.[26–32] However, the term cystadenocarcinoma was used loosely to encompass a subset of cases that likely represent papillary variants of secretory carcinoma, salivary duct carcinoma, or mucinous cystic variants of mucoepidermoid carcinomas.

Pathologic Features

IPMN presents as well-circumscribed uninodular, unicystic, or diffuse proliferations of the duct epithelium with a size range of 1 to 2.5 cm (see **Fig. 6**).[24] They show a prominent papillary growth of tall columnar mucinous epithelial cells arranged into 1 or multiple stratified layers along arborizing fibrovascular cores. The nuclei are basally located and rounded to oval or elongated with vesicular chromatin and conspicuous centrally located nucleoli. Mitotic figures are easily identified (ranging from 2 to 6 mitoses per high-power field).[24] Continuous or discontinuous involvement of most of the ductal system may be seen (see **Fig. 6**). Pale mucin-filled PAS-positive apical cytoplasmic droplets are seen and are reminiscent of gastric foveolar epithelium. However, no goblet cells, enterocytes, apocrine cells, oncocytes, squamoid cells, or any other cell type were seen. Necrosis and high-grade features were not observed. One case with foci of invasive micropapillary mucinous growth has been reported.[33]

By immunohistochemistry, IPMNs show uniform expression of CK7 but are negative for S100, androgen receptor, and p63. P63 highlights a discontinuous basal cell layer, but this may be

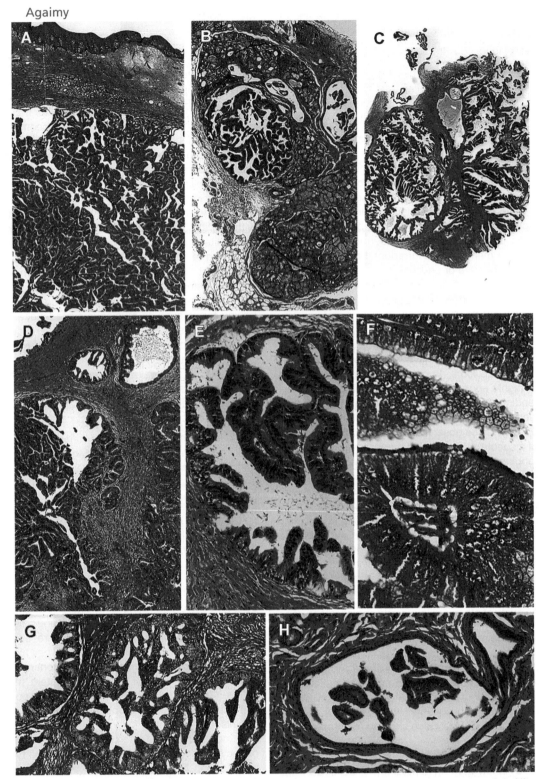

Fig. 6. Spectrum of IPMNs of the minor salivary glands. These uncommon tumors present as a unicystic nodule filling a dilated duct [hematoxylin-eosin, original magnification ×50] (*A*), involving more than 1 adjunct duct segments [hematoxylin-eosin, original magnification ×50] (*B*) or diffusely replacing the duct system resulting in prominent lobulation [hematoxylin-eosin, original magnification ×50] (*C*). (*D*) The architecture varies from simple or similar to atypical ductal hyperplasia of the breast (*upper field*) to highly complex confluent masses (*lower field*) [hematoxylin-eosin, original magnification ×100]. The cytologic features vary from intestinal-like [hematoxylin-eosin, original magnification ×200] (*E*) to gastric foveolar–like (*F*; note mitotic figure in the upper part) [hematoxylin-eosin, original magnification ×400]. Secondary cribriforming may be seen [hematoxylin-eosin, original magnification ×100] (*G*). (*H*) This microscopic intraluminal papillary lesion, which is similar to a few reports on ductal papillomas in the earlier literature, is part of the IPMN seen in (*B*) [hematoxylin-eosin, original magnification ×100].

Table 2
Proposed definition for intraductal papillary proliferations in the historical spectrum of ductal papillomas

Tumor Type	Main Features
Ductal papilloma, inverted	Well-circumscribed monomorphic papillary epidermoid growth
Ductal papilloma, exophytic	Exophytic-papillary monomorphic papillary epidermoid growth at ductal orifice
Intraductal papilloma	Papillary intraluminal growth, usually small[a]
IPMN, low grade	Prominent crowded complex papillary growth replacing a segment or involving diffusely the duct system, frequently with mucinous gastric-like epithelium, no frankly malignant cytologic features
IPMN, high grade	As above, but with frankly malignant cytologic features
IPMN, invasive[b]	As above; in addition, unequivocal invasion present[c]

Based on the recent WHO classification[1–3] and the current post-WHO literature.
  [a] Currently, there is no clear definition to separate intraductal papilloma from IPMN.
  [b] Specify extent of invasion and histologic subtype of invasive component.
  [c] The mere presence of extravasated mucus surrounding the cysts and the absence of a basal cell layer by immunohistochemistry do not indicate invasion.

absent and should not be mistaken for invasive growth.[13,24] The mucin profile was more akin to gastric foveolar epithelium, but data are limited by the small number of reported cases.[24]

Genetic Features of Salivary Gland IPMN

In the original report on salivary IPMN, all 3 neoplasms harbored the same substitution in the *AKT1* pleckstrin homology domain c.49G>A; p.Glu17Lys (E17K).[24] In a follow-up study by Nakaguro and colleagues,[13] 8 of 9 IPMNs showed the same *AKT1* mutation, thus confirming the previous report.[24] The 1 tumor without *AKT1* mutation harbored instead an *HRAS* Q61R mutation. Interestingly, 3 tumors harbored an *HRAS* Q61R in addition to the *AKT1* gene mutation, suggesting that the *HRAS* mutations may represent either an alternative driver event or possibly a second hit. Initial diagnoses of these IPMNs as papillary/cystadenoma (n = 2) and papillary/cystadenocarcinoma (n = 5) highlight the historical confusion of these papillary intraductal neoplasms and indicates that many have been misplaced in the cystadenoma or cystadenocarcinoma category.[13] Lack of similar mutation events in the 2 intraductal papillomas included points to the existence of distinct genetic entities on the spectrum of intraductal papillomas/IPMN, but more cases need to be examined before final conclusions can be drawn.

The protein kinase B (AKT) kinase isoforms AKT1, AKT2, and AKT3 are known downstream signaling effectors of the phosphatidylinositol 3-kinase (PI3K) pathway.[34] This molecular pathway is involved in manifold physiologic processes, such as cell metabolism, proliferation, and survival.[34] Oncogenic activation of the PI3K pathway is known to be tumorigenic and may result either from loss of inhibitory factors such as PTEN inactivation or from activating mutations in *PIK3CA* or *AKT*.[34] The *AKT1* E17K mutation has been reported in several neoplasms, including breast, colorectal, and ovarian cancers. Recently, the same mutation was reported in mammary ductal adenomas[35] and in anogenital hidradenoma papilliferum.[36] In the breast, the *AKT1* E17K mutation was detected in 54% of all papillomas, 15% of papillomas with hyperplasia, 27% of papillomas with atypical ductal hyperplasia, 43% of papillomas with carcinoma in situ, and in 10% of papillary carcinoma originating from a papilloma.[35] However, only very sparse data are available on the prevalence of the *AKT1* E17K mutation in salivary gland neoplasms (detected in 1.5% of salivary duct carcinoma).[37]

At present, it is not clear whether these IPMNs in the salivary glands do recapitulate their mammary counterpart or pancreatobiliary papillary mucinous neoplasms. Although the frequency of *AKT1* gene mutations is suggestive of a mammary analogue, the striking similarity of the IPMN of salivary glands to pancreatobiliary IPMN, occasionally to the extent that some have been mistaken for mucinous cystadenomas and mucinous cystadenocarcinomas, is more in line with a pancreatic-analogue lesion.[25] These neoplasms seem to show a greater tendency to recapitulate the gastric-type IPMN with frankly mucinous columnar epithelium that is distinct from other types of epithelia encountered in intercalated duct-type intraductal carcinoma, mucinous cystadenoma, and other types of ductal proliferative lesions of the salivary glands.

Prognosis and Treatment

Intraductal carcinoma with or without invasion have been reported to have originated from preexisting intraductal papillomas.[38–40] Recently, a case of salivary gland IPMN associated with invasive carcinoma was reported.[33] Accordingly, a classification scheme for these lesions analogous to their pancreatobiliary counterparts seems justified (see **Table 2**).

Differential Diagnosis

According to the literature, several cystic lesions with intraluminal papillary proliferations have likely been reported as papillary cystadenoma. Such misnamed lesions likely encompass both low-grade intercalated-type intraductal carcinoma and IPMN. As noted earlier in relation to cystadenomas, the presence of complex and arborizing branching papillae is unusual in cystadenoma and should justify consideration of intraductal carcinoma and IPMN. Admittedly, distinction of salivary IPMN from low-grade intraductal carcinoma based on current criteria is in some cases arbitrary. However, low-grade intraductal carcinoma is well definable by its phenotype, which recapitulates either the intercalated duct cells (S100, SOX10, and mammaglobin positive[7,19]) or, rarely, may show an apocrine phenotype.[41] A mixed intercalated-apocrine variant exists, although it is very rare, and it also harbors *RET* gene fusions.[7] The salivary IPMN cells are S100 negative, which enables their recognition and separation from the aforementioned cell types. Last but not least, salivary duct carcinoma with a mucinous component is a highly aggressive malignancy and should be separated from IPMN with invasion.[42]

CONFLICT OF INTEREST

None.

REFERENCES

1. Budnick S, Simpson RHW. Benign tumours of the salivary glands: Cystadenoma. In: El-Naggar AK, Chan JKC, Grandis JR, et al, editors. In: WHO classification of head and neck tumours. 4th edition. Lyon (France): IARC Press; 2017. p. 191.
2. Foschini MP, Bell D, Katabi N. Benign tumours of the salivary glands: Sialadenoma papilliferum. In: El-Naggar AK, Chan JKC, Grandis JR, et al, editors. In: WHO classification of head and neck tumours. 4th edition. Lyon (France): IARC Press; 2017. p. 192.
3. Richardson M, Bell D, Foschini MP, et al. Benign tumours of the salivary glands: ductal papillomas. In: El-Naggar AK, Chan JKC, Grandis JR, et al, editors. In: WHO classification of head and neck tumours. 4th edition. Lyon (France): IARC Press; 2017. p. 192–3.
4. Tjioe KC, de Lima HG, Thompson LD, et al. Papillary cystadenoma of minor salivary glands: report of 11 cases and review of the english literature. Head Neck Pathol 2015;9:354–9.
5. Stathopoulos P, Gagari E. Papillary cystadenoma of the lower lip exhibiting ciliated pseudostratified columnar epithelium: report of a bizarre case and review of the literature. Oral Maxillofac Surg 2013;17: 161–4.
6. Hernandez-Prera JC, Holmes BJ, Valentino A, et al. Macrocystic (Mammary Analogue) secretory carcinoma: an unusual variant and a pitfall in the differential diagnosis of cystic lesions in the head and neck. Am J Surg Pathol 2019;43:1483–92.
7. Skálová A, Ptáková N, Santana T, et al. NCOA4-RET and TRIM27-RET are characteristic gene fusions in salivary intraductal carcinoma, including invasive and metastatic tumors: is "intraductal" correct? Am J Surg Pathol 2019;43:1303–13.
8. Girotra C, Padhye MN, Mahajan P, et al. A rare case report of mucinous cystadenoma with immunohistochemical analysis and review of literature. J Maxillofac Oral Surg 2015;14(Suppl 1):426–34.
9. Sun S, Wang P, Wang Y, et al. Intraductal papilloma arising from the accessory parotid gland: a case report and literature review. Medicine (Baltimore) 2018;97:e10761.
10. Handra-Luca A. Mucinous cystadenoma of oral minor salivary glands: precursor of mucocele? Oral Oncol 2019;98:156–7.
11. Simionescu C, Florescu M, Margaritescu C, et al. Histopathologic and immunohistochemical study in one case of cystadenoma of parotid gland becoming malignant. Rom J Morphol Embryol 1999-2004;45:159–64.
12. Michal M, Skálová A, Mukensnabl P. Micropapillary carcinoma of the parotid gland arising in mucinous cystadenoma. Virchows Arch 2000; 437:465–8.
13. Nakaguro M, Urano M, Ogawa I, et al. Histopathological evaluation of minor salivary gland papillary-cystic tumours: focus on genetic alterations in sialadenoma papilliferum and intraductal papillary mucinous neoplasm. Histopathology 2020;76: 411–22.
14. Kakkar A, Zubair A, Sharma N, et al. Synchronous oncocytic papillary cystadenoma and warthin tumor

of the parotid gland. Int J Surg Pathol 2020;28(3): 296–301.

15. Stojanov IJ, Malik UA, Woo SB. Intraoral salivary duct cyst: clinical and histopathologic features of 177 cases. Head Neck Pathol 2017;11:469–76.

16. Fonseca FP, de Andrade BA, Lopes MA, et al. P63 expression in papillary cystadenoma and mucoepidermoid carcinoma of minor salivary glands. Oral Surg Oral Med Oral Pathol Oral Radiol 2013;115: 79–86.

17. Lanzel EA, Pourian A, Sousa Melo SL, et al. Expression of membrane-bound mucins and p63 in distinguishing mucoepidermoid carcinoma from papillary cystadenoma. Head Neck Pathol 2016; 10:521–6.

18. Skálová A, Vanecek T, Sima R, et al. Mammary analogue secretory carcinoma of salivary glands, containing the ETV6-NTRK3 fusion gene: a hitherto undescribed salivary gland tumor entity. Am J Surg Pathol 2010;34:599–608.

19. Weinreb I, Bishop JA, Chiosea SI, et al. Recurrent RET Gene Rearrangements in Intraductal Carcinomas of Salivary Gland. Am J Surg Pathol 2018; 42:442–52.

20. Seifert G. Mucoepidermoid carcinoma in a salivary duct cyst of the parotid gland. Contribution to the development of tumours in salivary gland cysts. Pathol Res Pract 1996;192:1211–7.

21. Brannon RB, Sciubba JJ, Giulani M. Ductal papillomas of salivary gland origin: a report of 19 cases and a review of the literature. Oral Surg Oral Med Oral Pathol Oral Radiol Endod 2001;92:68–77.

22. Aikawa T, Kishino M, Masuda T, et al. Intraductal papilloma arising from sublingual minor salivary gland: case report and immunohistochemical study. Oral Surg Oral Med Oral Pathol Oral Radiol Endod 2009;107:e34–7.

23. Ellis GL, Auclair PL. Intraductal papilloma. . Tumors of the salivary glands. Washington, D.C.: Armed Forces Institute of Pathology; 2008. p. 144–8.

24. Agaimy A, Mueller SK, Bumm K, et al. Intraductal papillary mucinous neoplasms of minor salivary glands with AKT1 p.Glu17Lys mutation. Am J Surg Pathol 2018;42:1076–82.

25. Furukawa T, Klöppel G, Volkan Adsay N, et al. Classification of types of intraductal papillary-mucinous neoplasm of the pancreas: a consensus study. Virchows Arch 2005;447:794–9.

26. Blanck C, Eneroth CM, Jakobsson PA. Mucus-producing adenopapillary [non-epidermoid] carcinoma of the parotid gland. Cancer 1971;28: 676–85.

27. Goldblatt LI, Ellis GL. Salivary gland tumors of the tongue. Analysis of 55 new cases and review of the literature. Cancer 1987;60:74–81.

28. de Araujo VC, de Sousa SO, Lopes EA, et al. Mucus producing adenopapillary carcinoma of minor salivary gland origin with signet ring cells and intracytoplasmic lumina. A light and electron microscopic study. Arch Otorhinolaryngol 1988;245:145–50.

29. Kardos TB, Ferguson JW, McMillan MD. Mucus-producing adenopapillary carcinoma of the oral cavity. Int J Oral Maxillofac Surg 1992;21:160–2.

30. Foss RD, Ellis GL, Auclair PL. Salivary gland cystadenocarcinomas. A clinicopathologic study of 57 cases. Am J Surg Pathol 1996;20:1440–7.

31. Pollett A, Perez-Ordonez B, Jordan RC, et al. High-grade papillary cystadenocarcinoma of the tongue. Histopathology 1997;31:185–8.

32. Aydin E, Turkoglu S, Ozen O, et al. Mucinous cystadenocarcinoma of a minor salivary gland in the upper lip: case report. Auris Nasus Larynx 2005;32:301–4.

33. Yang S, Zeng M, Chen X. Intraductal papillary mucinous neoplasm of the minor salivary gland with associated invasive micropapillary carcinoma. Am J Surg Pathol 2019;43:1439–42.

34. Carpten JD, Faber AL, Horn C, et al. A transforming mutation in the pleckstrin homology domain of AKT1 in cancer. Nature 2007;448:439–44.

35. Troxell ML, Levine J, Beadling C, et al. High prevalence of PIK3CA/AKT pathway mutations in papillary neoplasms of the breast. Mod Pathol 2010;23:27–37.

36. Goto K, Maeda D, Kudo-Asabe Y, et al. PIK3CA and AKT1 mutations in hidradenoma papilliferum. J Clin Pathol 2017;70:424–7.

37. Shimura T, Tada Y, Hirai H, et al. Prognostic and histogenetic roles of gene alteration and the expression of key potentially actionable targets in salivary duct carcinomas. Oncotarget 2017;9:1852–67.

38. Shiotani A, Kawaura M, Tanaka Y, et al. Papillary adenocarcinoma possibly arising from an intraductal papilloma of the parotid gland. ORL J Otorhinolaryngol Relat Spec 1994;56:112–5.

39. Kojima Y, Kano Y, Nagao K. Intraductal papillary adenocarcinoma of the submandibular gland. Otolaryngol Head Neck Surg 1998;118:404–7.

40. Nagao T, Sugano I, Matsuzaki O, et al. Intraductal papillary tumors of the major salivary glands: case reports of benign and malignant variants. Arch Pathol Lab Med 2000;124:291–5.

41. Bishop JA, Gagan J, Krane JF, et al. Low-grade apocrine intraductal carcinoma: expanding the morphologic and molecular spectrum of an enigmatic salivary gland tumor. Head Neck Pathol 2020. https://doi.org/10.1007/s12105-020-01128-0.

42. Tomihara K, Miwa S, Takazakura T, et al. Invasive micropapillary salivary duct carcinoma mixed with mucin-rich salivary duct carcinoma in minor salivary gland: a rare case report. Oral Surg Oral Med Oral Pathol Oral Radiol 2016;121:e162–7.

Myoepithelial Carcinoma

Bin Xu, MD, PhD, Nora Katabi, MD*

KEYWORDS

- Myoepithelial carcinoma • Carcinoma ex pleomorphic adenoma • Pleomorphic adenoma • *PLAG1*

Key points

- Myoepithelial carcinoma (MECA) may arise de novo or in association with a pleomorphic adenoma (carcinoma ex pleomorphic adenoma, CA ex PA).

- MECA can closely mimic pleomorphic adenoma (PA). The uniform cellular myoepithelial growth, the expansile nodular lobulated pattern, and the zonal cellular distribution may serve as useful diagnostic histologic features to differentiate MECA from PA.

- Compared with de novo MECA, CA ex PA correlates with worse clinical outcome.

- A grading system based on the presence of tumor necrosis should be used to identify high-grade MECA and predict its clinical behavior.

- MECA is a relatively aggressive tumor that is associated with a high rate of recurrence and distant metastasis.

ABSTRACT

Myoepithelial carcinoma (MECA) may overlap histologically with other salivary gland neoplasms, especially pleomorphic adenoma. MECA is characterized by cellular, uniform growth of myoepithelial cells and multinodular expansile invasive pattern with zonal cellular distribution. It may arise de novo or in association with pleomorphic adenoma (myoepithelial carcinoma ex pleomorphic adenoma). By immunohistochemistry, MECA is positive for cytokeratins and at least one of the myoepithelial markers, including S100. *PLAG1* fusion is the most common genetic alteration. Carcinoma ex pleomorphic adenoma and necrosis correlate with worse clinical outcome in MECA, and necrosis can be used to stratify MECA as high grade.

OVERVIEW

Myoepithelial carcinoma (MECA) is a malignant, infiltrative tumor that is composed almost exclusively of myoepithelial cells.[1,2] MECA was first described in the 1970s and was added to the second edition of the World Health Organization classification of salivary gland tumors in 1991.[1,3] It is a rare malignant salivary gland neoplasm that has been reported to comprise less than 2% of all salivary gland malignancies.[1,3] However, this tumor is underrecognized, and its incidence is currently thought to be higher.[3,4] The tumor may affect major and minor salivary glands, with the parotid gland being the most common location, followed by the palate and the submandibular gland.[1,5] MECA may arise de novo or in about 50% may develop in association with a preexistent pleomorphic adenoma (MECA ex PA).[1,2] It is the second most common histologic type of carcinoma ex PA, after salivary duct carcinoma.[2]

MECA affects both sexes equally.[1,2] MECA may happen at any age and has been reported in children.[5,6] Clinically, MECA has a diverse clinical outcome but seems to be relatively aggressive, especially in the setting of MECA ex PA even when it is intracapsular or minimally invasive.[3–5]

GROSS FEATURES

Grossly, MECA usually presents as an unencapsulated soft to firm mass with a gray to tan white cut

---

Department of Pathology, Memorial Sloan Kettering Cancer Center, 1275 York Avenue, New York, NY 10065, USA

* Corresponding author.
E-mail address: katabin@mskcc.org

Surgical Pathology 14 (2021) 67–73
https://doi.org/10.1016/j.path.2020.09.008

surgpath.theclinics.com

surface.[5] Necrosis, hemorrhage, and cystic and degenerative changes can be seen.[1,5]

MICROSCOPIC FEATURES

MECA is a histologically challenging entity, showing diverse morphologic features and heterogenous immunohistochemical findings.[3,4] The tumor is composed exclusively or almost exclusively of myoepithelial cells and exhibits an invasive growth pattern.[3,4] The neoplastic cells can be a mixture of cells, including spindled, epithelioid, plasmacytoid, vacuolated, and clear cells (**Fig. 1A–D**).[1,3,5–8] Regardless of the cell morphology, the myoepithelial cells often display a uniform monotonous cytology, perhaps reflecting the clonal growth of the malignant tumor. The tumor may exhibit solid, trabecular, or reticular patterns.[1,2,4,5,7] The stroma is myxoid and/or hyalinized.[1,2,4,5] Rarely, cartilaginous stroma may occur in MECA. Often the tumor displays a multinodular architecture with a lobulated uniformly cellular proliferation of myoepithelial cells and expansile pushing invasive borders[3,4] (**Fig. 2A**). A destructive invasive growth with infiltration into the adjacent structures is uncommon.[4] Zonal cellular arrangement consisting of hypercellular peripheral rim with hypocellular center is a common feature[3,4] (**Fig. 2B**), identified in greater than 50% of MECAs.[3] The hypocellular center might vary in volume and can be necrotic, myxoid, or hyalinized.[3,4] Occasionally, focal ductal formations and squamous differentiation can be seen.[1,3] The presence of tumor necrosis, CA ex PA, and vascular invasion were reported to correlate significantly with disease-free survival.[3]

TUMOR GRADING

There is no standard grading for MECA, and tumors with bland cytology and minimal mitotic activity have been reported to recur and cause death.[1,2,4,9,10] However, tumor necrosis was found to correlate with worse clinical behavior and can be used to identify high-grade MECA[3] (**Fig. 2C**).

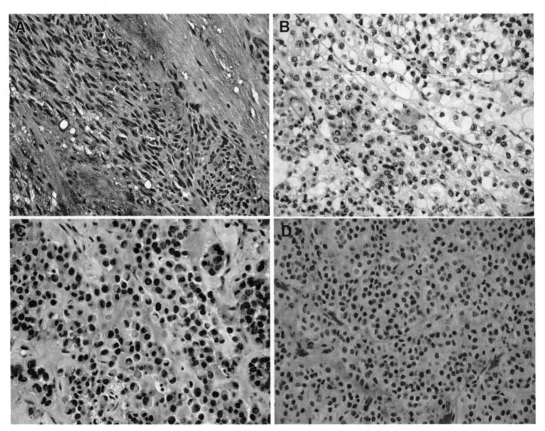

Fig. 1. Cytologic features of MECA. MECA can exhibit a mixture of cell types. (*A*) Spindle cells. (*B*) Clear cells. (*C*) Plasmacytoid cells. (*D*) Epithelioid cells.

Fig. 2. Histologic features of MECA. (*A*) MECA is characterized by uniform proliferation of myoepithelial cells with multinodular invasive pattern. (*B*) Zonal cellular distribution with a cellular periphery (P) and hypocellular (C) center is a common characteristic feature of MECA. (*C*) Necrosis (N) correlates with worse outcome and can be used to identify high-grade MECA.

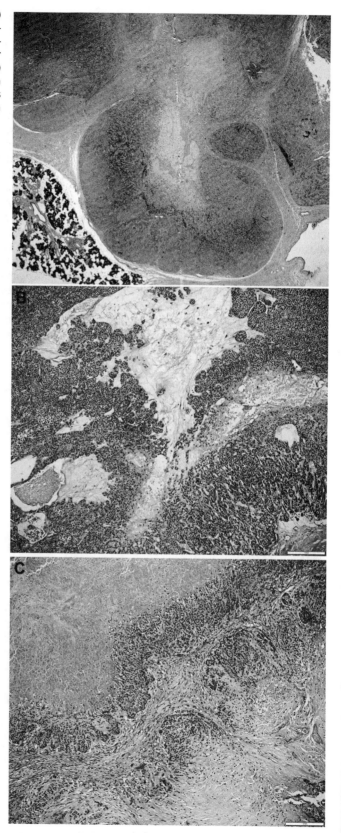

ANCILLARY STUDIES

IMMUNOHISTOCHEMISTRY

By immunohistochemistry, expression for a keratin and at least one of the myoepithelial markers is typically required to establish the diagnosis of MECA[1,3] (**Fig. 3**A–C). However, the tumor may exhibit a variable staining pattern for myoepithelial markers (**Table 1**).[3,4] A panel of several myoepithelial markers, including S100, smooth muscle actin (SMA), calponin, myosin, SOX10, glial fibrillary acidic protein (GFAP), p40, and p63, should be performed to confirm the myoepithelial differentiation in the tumor.[3,4,11,12] Although it is not entirely specific, S100 immunoexpression is identified in most MECAs (see **Fig. 3**B) and should be always included in their immunohistochemical panel.[3,4,9] PLAG1 immunohistochemical stain is a sensitive but not a specific marker of MECA ex PA and can be positive in other salivary neoplasms, such as PA and epithelial-myoepithelial carcinoma (**Fig. 3**D).[13] In addition, and despite the variable

immunostaining in MECA, immunohistochemistry can be helpful to highlight tumor architecture and identify the expansile lobulated nodular pattern within the tumor.[4]

MOLECULAR FEATURES

At the molecular level, *PLAG1* rearrangements are the most common genetic events identified in both de novo MECA and MECA ex PA and have been reported in 53% of the cases.[14–17] Furthermore, *TGFBR3-PLAG1* fusion was reported to be a potential specific marker for MECA, found in 15% of MECAs but not in PA or other salivary gland tumors.[14] *HMGA2* rearrangements were identified in about 10% of MECA.[14] Compared with de novo tumor, higher copy number alterations were identified in MECA ex PA, and this was found to correlate with poorer prognosis.[14] In addition to *PLAG1* fusion, *EWSR1* rearrangement was described in a subset of MECA that is composed mostly of clear myoepithelial cells and shows frequent necrosis.[18,19]

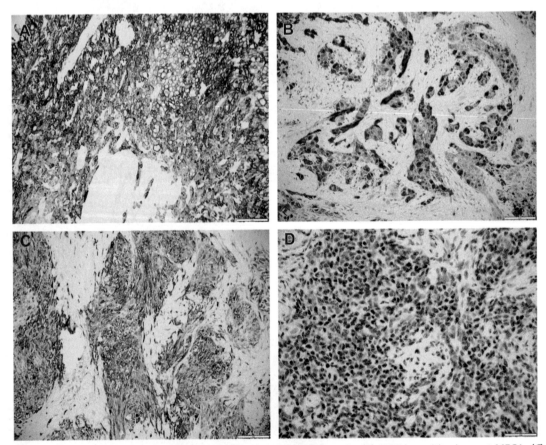

Fig. 3. Immunohistochemistry in MECA. (*A*) MECA is positive for keratin. (*B*) S100 is positive in most MECA. (*C*) Calponin staining in MECA. (*D*) PLAG1 showing nuclear staining in myoepithelial cells.

Table 1
Immunohistochemical stains in myoepithelial carcinoma

Immunohistochemistry	Percentage of Immunostaining
S100	89
Keratin	100
Calponin	76
SMA	64
p63	87.5

Adapted from Kong M, Drill EN, Morris L, et al. Prognostic factors in myoepithelial carcinoma of salivary glands: a clinicopathologic study of 48 cases. Am J Surg Pathol 2015;39(7):931-938; with permission.

DIFFERENTIAL DIAGNOSIS

PLEOMORPHIC ADENOMA

PA is the greatest mimic of MECA. Differentiating PA from MECA can be challenging, especially in cases of intracapsular or minimally invasive MECA ex PA and when high-grade features are absent.[1,3,4] The challenge to differentiate PA from MECA could be related to the difficulty in finding the malignant myoepithelial component, which may lead to misclassify the entire tumor as PA. The expansile lobulated multinodular myoepithelial growth and the zonal cellular distribution with hypercellular periphery and hypocellular are the 2 histologic features that help to distinguish MECA from PA (**Fig. 4**A–B). However, such features may not be evident in small material, for example, biopsy, rendering a definite distinction between these 2 entities difficult if not impossible.

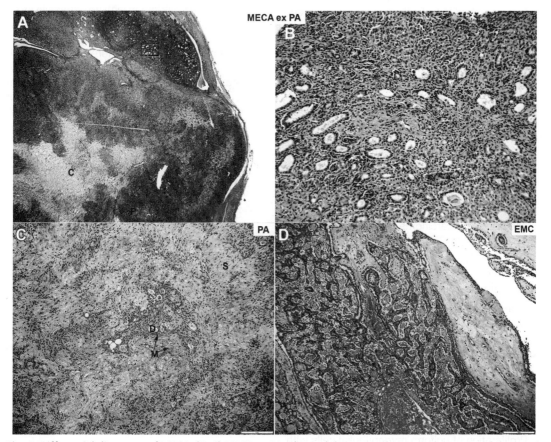

Fig. 4. Differential diagnoses of MECA. (*A, B*) MECA ex PA. The nodular expansile invasive pattern with hypercellular peripheral rim (P) and hypocellular center (C) in MECA ex PA helps to differentiate MECA from PA. (*B*) PA component of MECA ex PA (high power picture of the black box in *A*). (*C*) The typical heterogenous distribution of ducts (D), myoepithelial cells (M), and stroma (S) in PA. (*D*) EMC showing ductal cells surrounded by clear myoepithelial cells.

Moreover, the heterogenous arrangement of the ducts, myoepithelial cells, and stroma that is typically found in PA (**Fig. 4**C) along with the absence of the expansile myoepithelial growth can help to favor PA over MECA. Of note, satellite nodules or protrusions seen outside the PA capsule should be differentiated from the malignant nodular architecture of MECA. Furthermore, recurrent PA may display multiple tumor nodules mimicking the nodular pattern of MECA, but recurrent PA often presents as a miliary pattern of hypocellular myxoid nodules and shows a typical PA histology.

EPITHELIAL MYOEPITHELIAL CARCINOMA

True ducts can be found in MECA ex PA as part of the PA especially when the PA component in intermixed with the malignant myoepithelial component, and this should be distinguished from epithelial myoepithelial carcinoma (EMC). In contrast to de novo MECA in which true ducts are rare, the diagnosis of EMC should be considered if more than focal ducts are identified. Furthermore, MECA lacks the typical arrangement of EMC with ductal cells surrounded by multiple layer of myoepithelial cells often with clear cytoplasm (**Fig. 4**D).

MUCOEPIDERMOID CARCINOMA

Occasionally, focal squamous differentiation, myxoid stroma, and entrapped mucocytes in MECA may lead to misclassify MECA as mucoepidermoid carcinoma. The presence of abundant mucocytes and clear-cut epidermoid and intermediate cells along the negative staining for S100 and myoepithelial markers (ie, calponin and SMA) and the common *MAML2* fusion help to differentiate mucoepidermoid carcinoma from MECA.

POLYMORPHOUS ADENOCARCINOMA

Both MECA and polymorphous adenocarcinoma (PAC) may show myxoid stroma and one cell type and share similar immunohistochemical features. However, unlike MECA, PAC commonly exhibits a destructive infiltrative invasive pattern, a polymorphous diverse architecture, and frequent perineural invasion with targetoid arrangement around nerves and vessels.

DIAGNOSIS

1. Proliferation of uniform myoepithelial cells with invasive expansile nodular growth with pushing borders
2. Cellular zonal distribution of cells (ie, cellular peripheral rim and hypocellular center)

3. Immunohistochemical panel, including keratins, S100, and myoepithelial markers (calponin, SMA, GFAP, p63, and so forth)
4. PLAG1 fusions

PROGNOSIS

MECA has a diverse clinical behavior but seems to be relatively aggressive.[3,4,20,21] About one-third of patients experience recurrence, and one-third develop distant metastasis.[2,5] The tumor tends to have a propensity to distant metastasis rather than regional lymph node metastasis with lung being the most common site of distant metastasis.[3–5] Moreover, patients with MECA appear to have a nonnegligible risk of disease-related death of 13%.[4]

SUMMARY

MECA is a challenging entity and may be easily overlooked and misclassified. Cellular uniform myoepithelial proliferation with an expansile lobulated nodular pattern and zonal cellular distribution are characteristic of MECA and may serve as diagnostic histologic features to distinguish MECA from its mimics, especially PA. MECA can have adverse outcomes with a significant risk of distant and local recurrence even when it is intracapsular or minimally invasive MECA ex PA.

CLINICS CARE POINTS

- MECA is a relatively aggressive salivary gland tumor that is associated with high risk of recurrence and distant metastasis.

- The expansile lobulated multinodular myoepithelial growth and the zonal cellular distribution with hypercellular periphery and hypocellular center are the 2 histologic features that help to distinguish MECA from PA.

- Compared with de novo tumor, MECA ex PA correlates with worse clinical outcome.

- Necrosis is associated with worse behavior and can be used to identify high-grade MECA.

DISCLOSURE

The authors have nothing to disclose. Research reported in this publication was supported in part by the Cancer Center Support Grant of the National Institutes of Health/National Cancer Institute under award number P30CA008748. The content is solely the responsibility of the authors and does not necessarily represent the official views of the National Institutes of Health.

REFERENCES

1. Ellis GL, Auclair PL. Tumors of the salivary glands, vol Fascicle 9. Washington, DC: ARP Press; 2008.

2. Katabi N, Gomez D, Klimstra DS, et al. Prognostic factors of recurrence in salivary carcinoma ex pleomorphic adenoma, with emphasis on the carcinoma histologic subtype: a clinicopathologic study of 43 cases. Hum Pathol 2010;41(7):927–34.

3. Kong M, Drill EN, Morris L, et al. Prognostic factors in myoepithelial carcinoma of salivary glands: a clinicopathologic study of 48 cases. Am J Surg Pathol 2015;39(7):931–8.

4. Xu B, Mneimneh W, Torrence DE, et al. Misinterpreted myoepithelial carcinoma of salivary gland: a challenging and potentially significant pitfall. Am J Surg Pathol 2019;43(5):601–9.

5. El-Naggar AK, Chan JKC, Grandis JR, et al. World Health Organization classification of tumours: pathology and genetics of head and neck tumours. 4th edition. Lyon (France): International Agency for Research on Cancer (IARC); 2017.

6. Xu B, Aneja A, Ghossein R, et al. Salivary gland epithelial neoplasms in pediatric population: a single-institute experience with a focus on the histologic spectrum and clinical outcome. Hum Pathol 2017;67:37–44.

7. Barnes L. 3rd edition. Surgical pathology of the head and neck, vol 1. New York (NY): Informa Healthcare; 2009.

8. Di Palma S, Guzzo M. Myoepithelial carcinoma with predominance of plasmacytoid cells arising in a pleomorphic adenoma of the parotid gland. Histopathology 1998;33(5):485.

9. Kane SV, Bagwan IN. Myoepithelial carcinoma of the salivary glands: a clinicopathologic study of 51 cases in a tertiary cancer center. Arch Otolaryngol Head Neck Surg 2010;136(7):702–12.

10. Savera AT, Sloman A, Huvos AG, et al. Myoepithelial carcinoma of the salivary glands: a clinicopathologic study of 25 patients. Am J Surg Pathol 2000;24(6): 761–74.

11. Hsiao CH, Cheng CJ, Yeh KL. Immunohistochemical and ultrastructural study of malignant plasmacytoid myoepithelioma of the maxillary sinus. J Formos Med Assoc 1997;96(3):209–12.

12. Mendoza PR, Jakobiec FA, Krane JF. Immunohistochemical features of lacrimal gland epithelial tumors. Am J Ophthalmol 2013;156(6):1147–58.e1141.

13. Katabi N, Xu B, Jungbluth AA, et al. PLAG1 immunohistochemistry is a sensitive marker for pleomorphic adenoma: a comparative study with PLAG1 genetic abnormalities. Histopathology 2018;72(2):285–93.

14. Dalin MG, Katabi N, Persson M, et al. Multi-dimensional genomic analysis of myoepithelial carcinoma identifies prevalent oncogenic gene fusions. Nat Commun 2017;8(1):1197.

15. Katabi N, Ghossein R, Ho A, et al. Consistent PLAG1 and HMGA2 abnormalities distinguish carcinoma ex-pleomorphic adenoma from its de novo counterparts. Hum Pathol 2015;46(1): 26–33.

16. Martins C, Fonseca I, Roque L, et al. PLAG1 gene alterations in salivary gland pleomorphic adenoma and carcinoma ex-pleomorphic adenoma: a combined study using chromosome banding, in situ hybridization and immunocytochemistry. Mod Pathol 2005;18(8):1048–55.

17. Bahrami A, Dalton JD, Shivakumar B, et al. PLAG1 alteration in carcinoma ex pleomorphic adenoma: immunohistochemical and fluorescence in situ hybridization studies of 22 cases. Head Neck Pathol 2012;6(3):328–35.

18. Michal M, Skalova A, Simpson RH, et al. Clear cell malignant myoepithelioma of the salivary glands. Histopathology 1996;28(4):309–15.

19. Skalova A, Weinreb I, Hyrcza M, et al. Clear cell myoepithelial carcinoma of salivary glands showing EWSR1 rearrangement: molecular analysis of 94 salivary gland carcinomas with prominent clear cell component. Am J Surg Pathol 2015;39(3): 338–48.

20. Nagao T, Sugano I, Ishida Y, et al. Salivary gland malignant myoepithelioma: a clinicopathologic and immunohistochemical study of ten cases. Cancer 1998;83(7):1292–9.

21. Yang S, Li L, Zeng M, et al. Myoepithelial carcinoma of intraoral minor salivary glands: a clinicopathological study of 7 cases and review of the literature. Oral Surg Oral Med Oral Pathol Oral Radiol Endod 2010;110(1):85–93.

Lymphoepithelial Carcinoma of Salivary Glands

Lester D.R. Thompson, MD[a],*, Rumeal D. Whaley, MD[b]

KEYWORDS

- Lymphoepithelial carcinoma • Salivary gland • Immunohistochemistry • EBER

Key points

- Lymphoepithelial carcinoma is a rare undifferentiated primary salivary carcinoma that is associated with a florid lymphoid background.

- Epstein-Barr virus association is near 100% in endemic populations (e.g., Eskimo/Inuit) while the association in nonendemic populations is not as reproducible.

- Morphology, immunohistochemical stains, and Epstein-Barr virus encoded small RNA (EBER) in situ hybridization (ISH) are insufficient to distinguish lymphoepithelial carcinoma from nasopharyngeal carcinoma, which requires clinical evaluation.

- These tumors, irrespective of race or ethnicity, may express EBER, but a negative EBER-ISH does not exclude the diagnosis.

ABSTRACT

Lymphoepithelial carcinoma of salivary glands (LECSG) is an uncommon neoplasm. This article summarizes the findings of 438 cases in a review of the literature. Concurrent lymphoepithelial lesions may suggest a primary tumor. The tumor shows a nonkeratinizing carcinoma intimately associated with a rich lymphohistiocytic infiltrate, destroying adjacent salivary gland tissue. Irrespective of race or ethnicity, the tumors usually express Epstein-Barr virus, with Epstein-Barr virus encoded small RNA (EBER) and/or latent membrane protein-1 (LMP-1), although a subset does not. There is an overall good prognosis of about 80% at 5 years.

OVERVIEW

Undifferentiated carcinoma with an associated prominent, nonneoplastic, lymphoplasmacytic cell infiltrate is now called lymphoepithelial carcinoma (LEC).[1] It was originally described by Hilderman and colleagues[2] in 1962, as the possible malignant transformation of benign lymphoepithelial lesions (BLEL). LEC has gone by a diverse nomenclature, including but not limited to undifferentiated carcinoma, anaplastic parotid carcinoma, lymphoepitheliomalike carcinoma, lymphoepithelial-like carcinoma, undifferentiated carcinoma with lymphoid stroma, malignant lymphoepithelial lesion, nonnasopharyngeal undifferentiated carcinoma, and carcinoma ex lymphoepithelial lesion.[1,3–13] The historical names are not inherently inaccurate, but LEC most accurately reflects the intimate relationship between the epithelial and the lymphoid components of this neoplasm. Undifferentiated nasopharyngeal carcinoma (NPC) is the prototypical LEC.[8,14–16] It is most commonly reported in patients from Southeast Asian and Arctic Inuit populations, as well as descendants of these ethnic groups who migrate to nonendemic

a Department of Pathology, Southern California Permanente Medical Group, 5601 De Soto Avenue, Woodland Hills, CA 91365, USA; b IU Health Pathology Laboratory, Indiana University School of Medicine, 350 West 11th Street, Room 4014, Indianapolis, IN 46202, USA
* Corresponding author.
E-mail address: Lester.D.Thompson@kp.org
Twitter: @HeadandNeckPath (L.D.R.T.); Twitter: @RDWhaleyMD (R.D.W.)

Surgical Pathology 14 (2021) 75–96
https://doi.org/10.1016/j.path.2020.09.009
1875-9181/21/Published by Elsevier Inc.

countries.[17–19] Nearly all of the LECs in endemic patients express Epstein-Barr virus (EBV) in the neoplastic cells, which can be confirmed by a variety of different techniques. Within the salivary gland, LEC is rare, although it shows a strikingly high frequency in Arctic Inuit populations (Greenland, northern Canada, Alaska), southeastern Chinese, and Japanese, among others. Further, in Inuits especially, LEC of salivary gland (LECSG) is the most common salivary gland malignancy, mostly identified in the parotid gland. It accounts for up to 90% of all salivary gland malignancies.[4,5,8,9,12,20–24] It is always prudent to exclude a nasopharyngeal primary before making a definitive diagnosis of a salivary gland primary given similarly affected ethnic groups.[6,8,12]

CAUSE AND PATHOGENESIS

In almost all cases, the causal role of EBV is well documented, with EBV identified in the neoplastic epithelial cells by in situ hybridization or latent membrane protein 1 (LMP1) reactivity.[4–6,8,9,12,22,23,25–37] The neoplasm may progress as a malignant transformation of glandular or ductal inclusions in intraparotid gland lymph nodes or transformation of BLELs (epimyoepithelial islands),[3,12,38–46] although these structures may be reactive to the advancing tumor. There is clearly a complex interaction between genetic (ethnic), environmental, geographic, behavioral, and viral (EBV) factors in the oncogenic process of LEC.[6,47,48] Although there is a near-constant association of EBV with LEC in all ethnic groups, even in the salivary glands, it still must be recognized that EBV-negative LECs are documented in patients in nonendemic regions (**Table 1**).[49]

Most of the EBV-associated carcinomas are of the lymphoepithelial type. It may be that the active or vesicular nuclear appearance of the neoplastic cells is morphologically similar to the blastic transformation that occurs in EBV-infected B lymphocytes, suggesting that the lymphoid infiltrate may represent a host reaction to the virus-associated antigens that are expressed on the neoplastic cells.[50] Thus, an EBV infection seems to precede the oncogenic process, showing clonal episomal expansion.[51] Through a complex process, including EBV nuclear antigens and LMP1, EBV immortalizes B lymphocytes and prevents apoptosis.[52,53] Further, LMP1 in human epithelial cells has been shown to deregulate epithelial growth and inhibit differentiation, with the cells showing loss of contact inhibition, spindling, and a tendency to proliferate.[54] As such, the undifferentiated appearance may be caused by the role of LMP1.[6] Still sinonasal undifferentiated carcinoma shows a similar histologic appearance but is not EBV-associated. As such, the histologic appearance of LEC does not always indicate EBV association, nor is EBV association always associated with a lymphoepithelial pattern.[26] There is an increased risk of lymphoepithelial carcinomas (salivary or nasopharynx) in patients with human immunodeficiency virus (HIV) infection who progress to acquired immunodeficiency syndrome (AIDS).[55] However, HIV-associated salivary gland disease usually encompasses lymphoid hyperplasia, follicular involution, lymphoepithelial cysts (usually bilateral), and lymphoepithelial lesions.[56–59]

DEMOGRAPHICS

The incidence of a rare tumor is alwys difficult to estimate, and even more so when there is geographic diversity. As presented in **Table 2**, there is wide diversity in the incidence of LECSG in endemic regions, ranging from 0.3% to 54.8% of all tumors versus 3.6% to 92% of all malignant tumors.[9,11,20,34,37,60–64] By contrast, in nonendemic regions (see **Table 2**), the tumors represented 0.3% to 0.7% of all malignant tumors.[47,65] Higher incidences of LEC are reported in Arctic region natives (Eskimos/Inuits from Alaska, Canada, Greenland), southern Chinese, Japanese, northern Africans, and Mongolians.[4,6,21,22,37,66] Of these endemic populations, the Eskimo/Inuit population seems to be the most affected.[11,32] When white people are included in the published cases, they represent about 7% of all reported cases, although higher numbers (62%) are found in nonendemic reports.[49]

Individual case series have shown a sex bias, even when endemic considerations are taken into account. However, when all reported cases are aggregated, there is no sex predilection (see **Table 1**).

Patients of a wide age range are affected, from 10 to 86 years, with a mean of 47.1 years and a median of 46.0 years. However, nonendemic patients tend to be older (mean, 55.4 years; median, 55 years).[25,28,33,35,36,47,49,55,67–69]

CLINICAL FINDINGS

Given the rarity of LECSG, clinical findings are difficult to extrapolate, but patients present with nonspecific symptoms, including swelling or a mass in the salivary gland (**Fig. 1**), with pain (approximately 5%) and nerve findings (approximately 2.5%) uncommonly recognized.[5,60,66] In

Table 1
Literature summary of 438 patients with lymphoepithelial carcinomas of salivary gland

Characteristics[a]	Number (n = 438)
Sex	
Female	210
Male	211
Age (y)	
Range	10–86
Mean	47.1
Median	46.0
Ethnicity	
Asian	321
Inuit/Eskimo/Native Canadian Indian	49
White	40
Black	6
Middle East	1
Symptom Duration (mo)	
Range	0.5–240
Mean	20.8
Median	11.5
Clinical Presentation	
Swelling/mass	413
Pain	21
Nerve paralysis/paresis	14
Site	
Parotid	333
Submandibular gland	75
Sublingual gland	2
Minor salivary gland	26
Palate	17
Laterality	
Left	35
Right	44
Tumor Size (cm)	
Range	0.7–15
Mean	3.9
Median	3.8
Women (mean, cm)	4.4
Men (mean, cm)	3.6
White (mean, cm)	4.2
Inuits/Eskimos and Asians (mean, cm)	3.8
Black (mean, cm)	4.2
Epstein-Barr virus encoded small RNA Status	
Positive	265
Negative	16

(continued on next column)

Table 1
(continued)

Characteristics[a]	Number (n = 438)
Lymph node metastasis identified	73
Therapy	
Surgery (including neck dissection)	389
Surgery and radiation	156
Surgery, radiation, and chemotherapy	20
Patients with follow-up (n = 141) (mean months of follow-up)	
Alive, no evidence of disease	106 (63.3)
Alive with disease	8 (53.5)
Dead, no evidence of disease	5 (32.3)
Dead of disease	22 (40.4)
Follow-up (mo)	
Range	2–303
Mean	57.7

[a] Not stated in all cases.
Data from Refs.[2,4–10,12,13,20,21,23–28,30–40,43,49,60,66,67,69,74–78,80,82,84–88,121,129,137–139,141–160]

advanced cases, skin and soft tissue fixation may be seen. Symptoms are present over an exceptionally broad time frame, ranging from 0.5 to 180 months, although most patients report slightly less than 2 years of symptoms, with a median of 11.5 months. Clinically or radiographically obvious cervical lymphadenopathy is detected in about 17% of patients (see **Table 1**). Almost all tumors affect the major glands, with the parotid (76%) and submandibular glands (17%) accounting for 93% of all tumors. Minor salivary gland sites are uncommon, but, when identified, the palate accounts for approximately 65% of all tumors. On imaging, patients show a partially circumscribed or ill-defined mass with a lobular or plaquelike lesion (**Fig. 2**), with homogeneous to heterogeneous enhancement. Occasionally, intratumoral necrosis or cystic change is noted. Soft tissue invasion into adjacent structures is common, along with radiographically involved cervical lymph nodes.[60,70–73]

LABORATORY STUDIES

Most patients show some serologic evidence of previous infection with EBV. Although EBV viral capsid antigen (VCA) to immunoglobulin (Ig) A, IgM, and/or IgG, EBV nuclear antigen (EBNA)

Table 2
Lymphoepithelial carcinomas of salivary gland incidence variation

Cohort Reported	Number of LECSG Cases	All Salivary Gland Tumors[a]	Total Number of Malignant Salivary Gland Tumors	Cases
Endemic Population				
Arthaud,[9] 1972	7	19	NR	36.8% of all tumors
Nielsen et al,[11] 1978	23	42	25	54.8% of all tumors 92% of malignant tumors
Nagao et al,[37] 1996	5	1676	NR	0.3% of all tumors
Saku et al,[20] 2003	162 total 124 southern China only	NR	4330 (at least) 1965 southern China only	3.7% of all malignant tumors 6.3% of southern China only
Wang et al,[60] 2004	16	NR	295	5.4% of malignant tumors
Zhang et al,[61] 2005	16	NR	444	3.6% of all malignant tumors
Li et al,[62] 2008	52	3461	1392	1.5% of all tumors 3.7% of all malignant tumors
Tian et al,[63] 2010	121	6982	2239	1.7% of all tumors 5.4% of all malignant tumors
Wang et al,[64] 2012	28	1176	289	2.4% of all tumors 9.7% of malignant tumors
Li et al,[34] 2014	50	NR	235	21.3% of malignant tumors
Nonendemic Population				
Jones et al,[65] 2008 (United Kingdom)	1	741	260	0.1% of all tumors 0.3% of all malignant tumors
Zhan et al,[47] 2016 (United States)	238	NR	36,224	0.66% of all malignant tumors

Abbreviation: NR, not reported.
[a] Major and/or minor salivary gland sites.

IgG, and early antigen (EA)-IgG antibodies are seen in patients with a past infection, they are not always seen in patients with LEC.[32] It is interesting that sometimes these findings precede the documentation of LEC. However, levels of IgA antibodies to EBV VCA are usually increased in patients with carcinoma.[74]

CYTOLOGY

Smears show single to clustered large polygonal and spindled cells in syncytial sheets. The cells have limited to moderate amounts of cytoplasm and have a high-grade, undifferentiated appearance (**Fig. 3**). The nuclei are vesicular with prominent nucleoli. Mitotic activity is brisk. Most have a prominent mixed lymphoid population that may mask the isolated epithelial elements, resulting in a misdiagnosis.[69,75–78] Metastatic nasopharyngeal carcinoma to an intra–salivary gland lymph node may also be a consideration. Further, a dense lymphoplasmacytic infiltrate may mimic an intra–salivary gland lymph node, and, depending on the type of population present, may suggest a lymphoma. If the epithelial cells are not atypical, lymphoepithelial sialadenitis or lymphoepithelial cyst

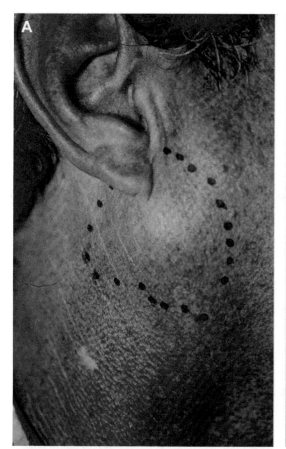
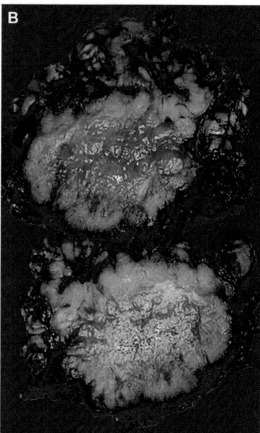

Fig. 1. (*A*) Clinical examination showed a parotid gland swelling without skin erythema in a patient without a nasopharyngeal mass. (*B*) There is a fish-flesh pale cut surface of the parotid gland, showing a mass replacing the entire gland.

may also be considered. Many primary salivary gland neoplasms have a prominent lymphoid stroma associated with them, such as mucoepidermoid carcinoma and acinic cell carcinoma, and these tumors should not be confused with LEC. If cell block material is available, especially in endemic patients, EBER may aid in separation between the epithelial lesions and even lymphomas that are EBV associated.

MACROSCOPIC FEATURES

LECSGs grossly are typically circumscribed but not encapsulated, with a lobulated, firm, tan-white cut appearance (see **Fig. 1**). Other cases show an infiltrative appearance into the adjacent salivary glands, fat, skeletal muscle, and skin. The tumors range up to 15 cm,[16,47,69] with most greater than 2 cm.

MICROSCOPIC FEATURES

Although the histologic features are characteristic and identical to nonkeratinizing nasopharyngeal carcinoma, it is important to recognize that variability in amount and type of epithelial elements may be present, along with the amount and type of lymphoid infiltrate (sparse to heavy). Original descriptions suggested malignant transformation from lymphoepithelial sialadenitis (LESA) or myoepithelial sialadenitis (MESA).[8,16,35,46,56,79–81] Thus, in some cases, it is possible that LESA may be seen adjacent to or even within the tumor (**Fig. 4**), a finding that favors a primary tumor rather than a metastatic lesion. It may be that LESA is a reaction rather than a precursor, but a precursor is favored. However, there are investigators who do not agree that LESA or MESA is seen in or adjacent to these tumors.[6] There does not seem to be an

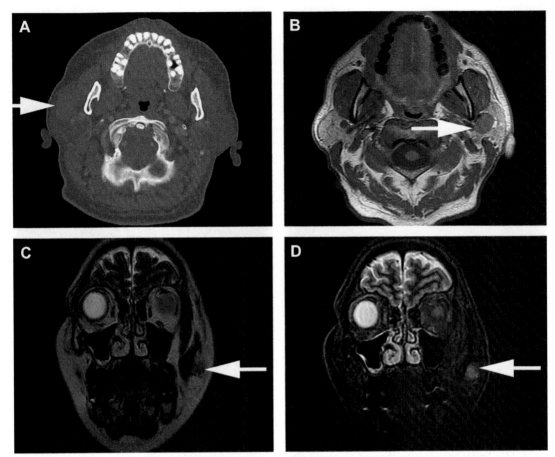

Fig. 2. LEC affecting the: (*A*) Right parotid gland as a soft tissue swelling (*arrow*) by axial computed tomography; (*B*) A left parotid gland well-defined hypointense mass (*arrow*) on T1-weighted axial magnetic resonance (MR); (*C*) A hypointense mass (*arrow*) on coronal T2-weighted MR; and (*D*) Hyperintense mass on coronal T2-STIR (short T1 inversion recovery) sequence MR (*arrow*).

association with autoimmune disorders (e.g., Sjögren disease).[16,46,49,56,74] In classic form, the epithelial component shows a syncytium of crowded, large, undifferentiated cells with a high nuclear to cytoplasmic ratio; irregular to geometric or oval nuclei; vesicular to open nuclear chromatin; and large, prominent, brightly hypereosinophilic nucleoli (**Fig. 5**). The cytoplasm is sparse, delicate, and lightly staining. Smudged nuclei may be seen within some of the neoplastic cells (see **Fig. 5**). Pleomorphism in the nuclei is often easily recognized (**Fig. 6**).[60,66,74] Definitive squamous differentiation, including keratinization, may be present (see **Fig. 6**), although usually limited in extent, whereas tumor cell spindled and even a basaloid morphology can be identified, resulting in some patients showing a hybrid morphology.[82] In general, the adjacent salivary gland tissue is unremarkable, lacking any prominent lymphoid infiltration (see **Fig. 6**).

All tumors are infiltrative by definition, frequently expanding beyond the salivary gland parenchyma into the adjacent soft tissues, and even showing positive surgical margins in about a quarter of patients.[47] Two major patterns of growth are recognized, described by their eponyms, named after the German pathologist Alexander Schmincke (1877–1953) and French radiologist Claude Regaud (1870–1941), who researched this tumor type and independently reported their cases in the same year.[20] The Schmincke-type pattern shows syncytial clusters of undifferentiated tumor cells in an intimate relationship with the lymphoid cells and seemingly overrun by them (**Fig. 7**), making it challenging to detect the epithelial cells. The Regaud-type shows sheets, cords, and cohesive nests that are set within and even separated by the lymphoid stroma, which may contain germinal centers, usually showing epithelial groups well circumscribed and distinct from the adjacent

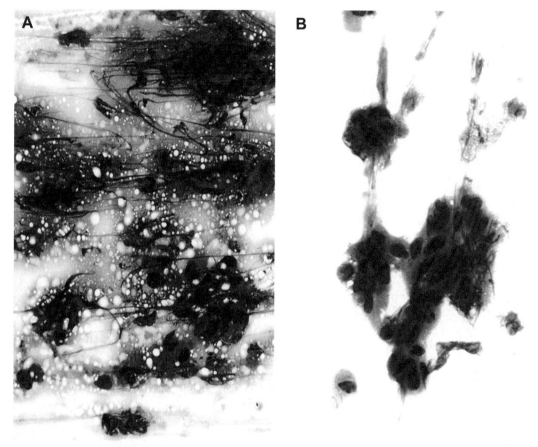

Fig. 3. (A) The smears are cellular, showing prominent lymphoid matrix tangles in the background with large, polygonal, syncytial epithelial cells (air dried, May-Grüwald–Giemsa [MGG]). (B) There is a cluster of atypical epithelial cells with a high nuclear to cytoplasmic ratio (air dried, MGG).

parenchyma (**Fig. 8**). It is common to have the islands resemble a jigsaw puzzle (see **Fig. 8**). Mitoses are easily identified and include atypical forms. Tumor necrosis is usually not a prominent finding (see **Fig. 8**), except in the basaloid LEC. The lymphoid stroma is rich, containing a nearly equal number of polyclonal B and T lymphocytes and plasma cells. Germinal center formation is frequently identified (i.e., nonneoplastic lymphoid elements). The reactive histiocytes within the lymphoid compartment can be prominent, yielding a starry-sky appearance (**Fig. 9**). Importantly, there is nothing to suggest the formation of a true lymph node: no medullary zone, no subcapsular sinus or sinus histiocytosis, and no cortical zone. This finding can be confirmed by performing CAM5.2 immunohistochemistry, which highlights extrafollicular reticulum cells seen in a true lymph node.[83] Noncaseating granulomatous inflammation along with multinucleated giant cells may be seen, either as a reaction to the neoplastic cells

or to debris (see **Fig. 9**). Amyloid in the form of extracellular, acellular, eosinophilic matrix material may be seen, sometimes surrounded by the neoplastic cells.[2,5,24,49,74] There is usually an absence of stromal reaction in the form of desmoplasia, a finding frequently seen in other types of salivary gland neoplasm. Salivary gland ducts, glands, and acini may be seen at the periphery of the tumor, occasionally entombed.

Squamous differentiation is usually not the dominant finding, but areas of squamous differentiation can be seen. When present, a metastatic neoplasm to the salivary gland and/or lymph nodes must be considered.[16,74] Tumor cell spindling may be prominent (**Fig. 10**), resulting in a fascicular pattern, sometimes with desmoplastic stroma. This finding brings to mind other tumor categories such as basal cell adenoma and myoepithelial carcinoma, among others.[16,35,37,40,45] Rare cases of epithelial-myoepithelial carcinoma may be EBV associated, highlighting a

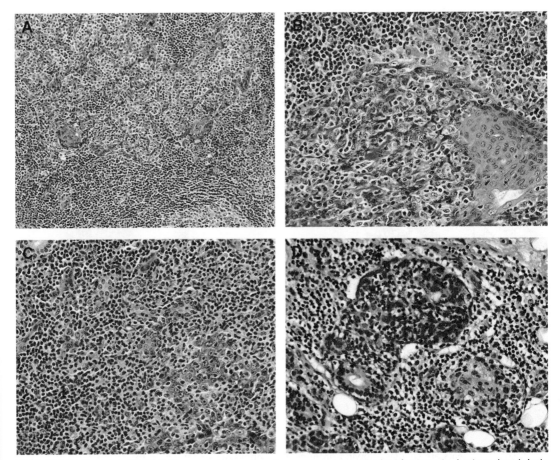

Fig. 4. LESA adjacent to LEC. (*A*) Monocytoid lymphocytes are seen associated with a terminal acinar duct lobule. (*B*) Squamous metaplasia intimately associated with lymphoid elements. (*C*) Epithelial proliferation associated with lymphocytes, but lacking cytologic atypia. (*D*) A terminal duct with inflammatory cells. Histiocytes are noted in the lower right corner.

transformation from the benign spindled cells of an MESA to LEC.[84] The basaloid morphology has been described primarily in Inuit populations, with a consistent EBV association identified,[82] showing a sclerotic stroma, limited lymphoid tissue, and angulated cord or "syringoma-like" nests. Perineural invasion may be prominent (see **Fig. 10**). Importantly, a cutaneous basal cell carcinoma must be eliminated, because they may directly invade into the parotid salivary gland.

ULTRASTRUCTURAL FINDINGS

Although almost never used in the twenty-first century, it is important to recognize the findings on electron microscopy, because they underpin the diagnosis. The tumor cells are usually closely apposed and joined by well-developed desmosomes (although in limited numbers). The nuclei are large, slightly irregular, with peripheral condensation of heterochromatin and large, single, central nucleoli. Spherical fibrillary nuclear bodies may be seen in the neoplastic cells but not in the lymphocytes. The cytoplasm contains a variable number of bundles of tonofilaments. Lymphocytes can be seen intimately associated with the neoplastic cells.[31,40,45,77,85,86] Importantly, no secretory lumina or vacuoles or tight junctions are seen.

IMMUNOHISTOCHEMISTRY AND IN SITU HYBRIDIZATION FINDINGS

LECSGs are epithelial neoplasms, and thus are highlighted with a variety of markers of epithelial differentiation, to include pancytokeratin, AE1/AE3 (**Fig. 11**), CAM5.2, CK903, CK5/6 (see **Fig. 11**), and epithelial membrane antigen (EMA), along with p40 and p63 (**Fig. 12**).[5,16,20,30,49,87,88] The reactivity may be strong and diffuse, or yield

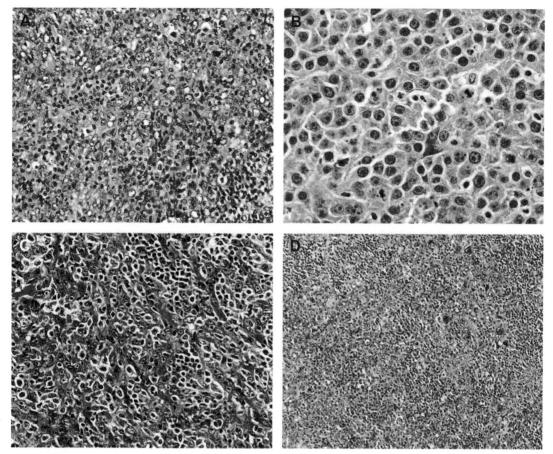

Fig. 5. Cellular features of LEC. (*A*) Syncytium of large, polygonal neoplastic cells with vesicular chromatin. (*B*) Large, prominent, hypereosinophilic nucleoli. (*C*) Cytoplasmic extensions surround vesicular nuclei. (*D*) Smudge and focal tumor giant cells within a sea of neoplastic cells.

a more characteristic lace-like or lattice-like wispy staining of the delicate cytoplasmic extensions that are pushed by the inflammatory infiltrate (see **Fig. 11**). SOX10 may highlight basaloid-type cells,[89] whereas dendritic cells are highlighted with S100 protein. CD117 is noted in some cases, but p16 and high-risk human papillomavirus (HPV) by in situ hybridization (ISH) are negative.

Considered to be most helpful, especially in separating from other neoplasms in the salivary gland, is the strong and diffuse reactivity with either a membranous and granular cytoplasmic EBV LMP1 pattern or a nuclear EBER by ISH (see **Fig. 12**), the latter confirming the presence of the EBV-encoded small RNAs (EBERs).[4,6,20,25,29,37,40,48,49,69] The EBER signals are often localized to the perinucleolar area and along the nuclear membrane. Of course, no signals are identified in the adjacent lymphocytes. Although these EBV studies confirm the diagnosis in endemic populations, they are not always seen in nonendemic populations (see **Table 1**). Thus, the absence of EBV in LEC suggests that other factors (e.g., environmental and genetic predisposition) may also contribute to the pathogenesis of the tumor.[4,35,48,49,67,78]

POLYMERASE CHAIN REACTION AMPLIFICATION AND DNA SEQUENCING

Not routinely performed, polymerase chain reaction (PCR) amplification of LMP1 shows that the 30-bp deleted variant (from the C-terminal region of the EBV LMP1 gene) is the most consistently identified within tumors found in patients from the endemic areas. Point mutations in codons 322 (Gln to Asn) and 334 (Gln to Arg) are found in nearly all tested patients, along with mutations in codons 335 and 338, suggesting highly shared mutations in EBVs seen in salivary gland LEC, findings similar to those reported in nasopharyngeal

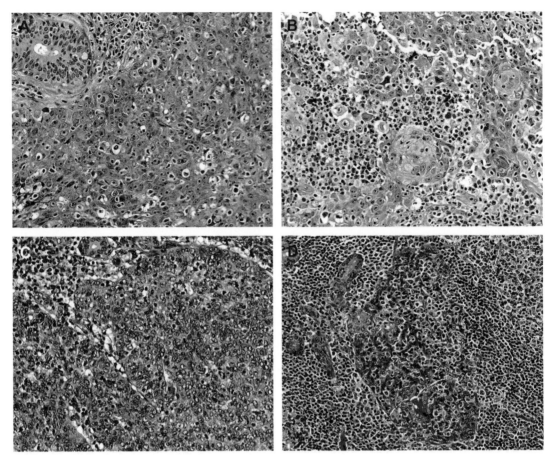

Fig. 6. (*A*) Cellular pleomorphism is easily noted, with a benign duct for comparison. (*B*) Keratin pearl formation is seen, along with an acute inflammatory infiltrate. (*C*) Adjacent ducts are unremarkable, with tumor arranged in a sheet. (*D*) There is subtle atypia in this central island of tumor, adjacent to a duct and a germinal center.

carcinomas.[90] In most patients, the EBV is specific to the tumor, documented by a strong EBER in the nuclei of the neoplastic cells, but completely lacking in the adjacent normal or uninvolved tissues.[6,32]

DIFFERENTIAL DIAGNOSIS

The histologic appearance of LECSG should bring to mind a variety of undifferentiated lesions that develop in the salivary gland, along with tumors that have a rich inflammatory infiltrate. Depending on the proportions of each element, the differential diagnosis may be different.

When the lymphoid component is dominant, a lymphoepithelial lesion, reactive tumor-associated lymphoid proliferation (TALP), lymphadenoma, Warthin tumor, and lymphoma are all brought to the fore. LESA lacks a destructive infiltration, maintaining a lobular appearance,[56,91] and may have associated clinical and laboratory features of Sjögren syndrome. The lymphoid component can be prominent in these lesions, partly obscuring the epithelial islands, with remnants of the glandular and ductal epithelium seen scattered in the background. However, the ducts and acini affected with LESA do not become cytologically atypical, and lack overt cytomorphologic features of malignancy, showing epithelial and myoepithelial cells within more characteristic patterns, frequently showing squamous metaplasia. LESA or BLEL do not show EBER or LMP1 reactivity, a finding that helps with separation from the EBV-associated LECSG. Clinically, a rapidly enlarging mass over a few weeks favors carcinoma. Clearly in EBV-unassociated LECSG, this test would not be useful. Chronic sclerosing sialadenitis shows marked sclerosing fibrosis, a rich plasma cell infiltration with parenchymal atrophy, known to be part of IgG_4-sclerosing disease.[92] TALP is commonly encountered in acinic cell carcinoma and in mucoepidermoid carcinoma, and

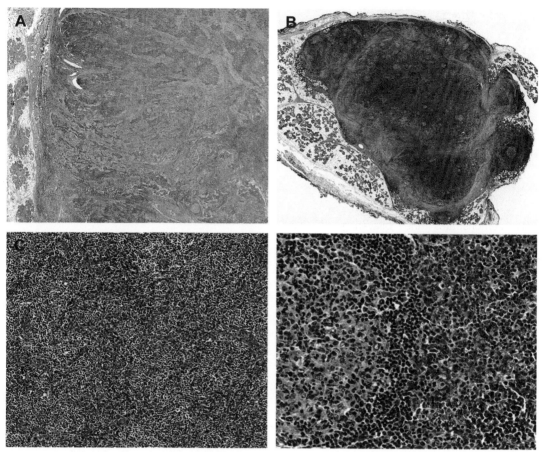

Fig. 7. Classic Schmincke pattern. (*A*) Circumscribed tumor, arranged in sheets with separating fibrosis. (*B*) Multi-nodular tumor with prominent lymphoid component, showing numerous germinal centers. (*C*) Subtle epithelial component intermixed with the lymphoid cells. (*D*) A germinal center (*left*) as a point of comparison for the neoplastic cells (*right*).

less commonly in lymphoepithelial cystadenocarcinoma. The epithelial elements of an acinic cell carcinoma tend to be more cohesive, lack a syncytial architecture, lack vesicular nuclear chromatin, and usually have cytoplasmic, dark blue zymogen granules.[93–96] The epithelial cells are DOG1, SOX10, and NR4A3 immunoreactive, findings that are not seen in LECSG.[97] Mucoepidermoid carcinoma, especially if higher grade, may have some similarities in growth. However, the transitional epithelium and mucinous differentiation are findings not identified in LEC. The immunohistochemistry findings might be similar (CK-pan, CK5/6, p40, p63), and so, in some instances, a *MAML2* fluorescence in situ hybridization (FISH) evaluation may be the only definitive way to make a separation.[98–102] Lymphadenoma, sebaceous lymphadenoma, and lymphadenocarcinoma (often cystic) are tumors associated with a rich lymphoid infiltrate where the epithelial cells

are basaloid, squamous, and glandular, forming solid nests, cords, tubules, and cysts. Sebaceous differentiation is seen in some of these tumors, whereas malignant transformation is rare. In lymphadenoma, the tumors are well defined, lack infiltration, and lack cytologic atypia. There is an even distribution of the epithelial elements within the lymphoid stroma. The tumor cells are negative with EBV markers.[103–105] A Warthin tumor must show oncocytically altered epithelium, usually in a characteristic bilayered, tram-track appearance, with cysts and papillary structures, associated with a rich inflammatory infiltrate. There is no pleomorphism, no vesicular nuclear chromatin, and a lack of EBER.[56,106–108] Although rarely an EBV-associated diffuse large B-cell lymphoma may be seen in a Warthin tumor,[109–111] generally the lymphomas of the salivary gland are either extranodal marginal zone B-cell lymphomas (which are not EBV associated) or diffuse large B-cell

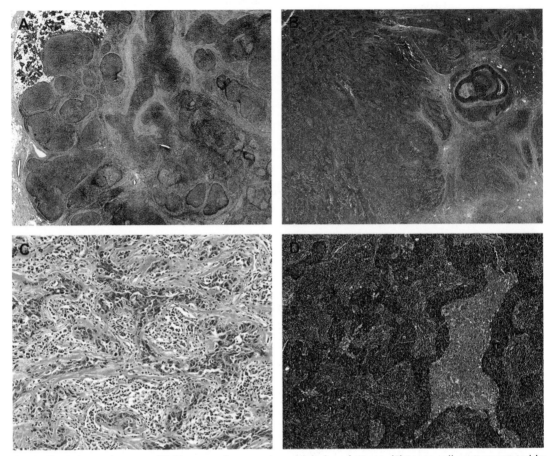

Fig. 8. Classic Regaud pattern (*A*) There are large nests and lobules of tumor. (*B*) Large cell nests separated by heavy fibrosis, creating a jigsaw appearance. (*C*) High-power view of a jigsaw pattern with a more prominent stroma. (*D*) Central area of comedonecrosis surrounded by ribbons of neoplastic cells.

lymphomas, some of which may be EBV associated.[56,112–118] In such cases, the lack of any epithelial markers in a sheetlike tumor population that destroys the native salivary gland parenchyma, and in which it is the lymphoid cells that are reactive with EBV, among other lymphoid markers, can help to confirm a lymphoma diagnosis (including Hodgkin lymphoma).[113,116,119,120]

When the epithelial cells predominate, an undifferentiated or high-grade transformation that may be seen in some primary salivary gland neoplasms and metastatic tumors must be excluded. The most important distinction when LEC is considered is to exclude a metastasis from a nasopharyngeal primary. The highest incidence of NPC is in the same endemic group of patients with the highest incidence of LECSG, and both are EBV associated to a very high degree. As such, clinical, endoscopic, imaging, and even biopsy findings of the nasopharynx must be incorporated to exclude

this possibility, with many of the case reports and clinical series in the literature documenting these findings.[4,6,9,10,12,16,21,26,31–33,35,37,38,47,60,74,77,78, 88,121] Rarely, a lymphoepithelial pattern may be seen in oropharyngeal squamous cell carcinoma (SCC), usually HPV associated, and salivary gland metastasis may be seen. A strong, diffuse, nuclear, and cytoplasmic p16 reaction in more than 70% of the neoplastic cells and/or ISH for high-risk HPV may be helpful in this setting to confirm an oropharyngeal primary.[122–124] Especially when poorly differentiated, SCC may present as metastatic disease to the parotid gland and lymph nodes. The tumors may not be keratinizing and may have a morphologic appearance that is identical to LEC when presenting in a lymph node. However, most metastatic SCCs to salivary glands are from skin primaries, whereas mucosal primaries are much less common. Skin primaries are not EBER reactive, but are difficult to separate

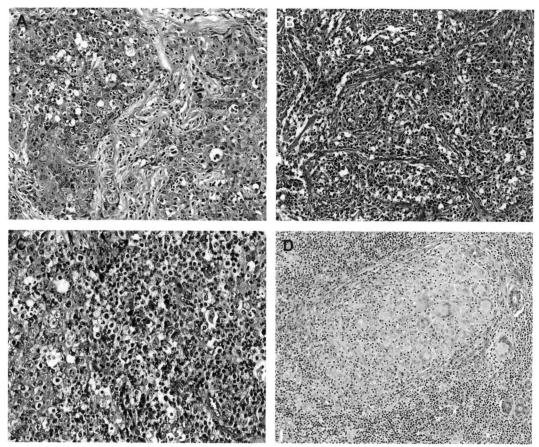

Fig. 9. (*A*) Starry-sky appearance is composed of both lymphocytes and epithelial cells. (*B*) Numerous histiocytic cells create a starry-sky appearance. (*C*) Neoplastic cells adjacent to areas of acute inflammation and histiocytes. (*D*) Multinucleated giant cells with histiocytes are present adjacent to the tumor.

in EBV-negative LECSG. Careful clinical correlation with known skin or mucosal primary SCC must be achieved. NUT carcinoma is exceptionally rare in salivary gland (primary or metastatic), showing poorly cohesive small to medium-sized cells with abrupt and focal squamous differentiation, and must show NUT immunohistochemical reactivity.[125] Adamantinoma-like Ewing sarcoma may be primary in the salivary gland but tend to show a basaloid morphology, infiltrative growth, and nuclear monotony, and tend not to have overt keratinization, while showing CD99 and NKX2.2 reactivity but lacking EBER.[126,127] Poorly differentiated carcinomas of the salivary gland are primary carcinomas that include a large cell undifferentiated category, in addition to neuroendocrine carcinomas. Large cell undifferentiated carcinoma (lacks evidence of glandular, squamous, or neuroendocrine differentiation) has an organoid growth, minimal differentiation, high mitotic rate, and coagulative necrosis, but lacks the lymphoid

infiltrate and, by definition, lacks EBV.[60,128–130] Thus, in EBV-negative LECSG, the lack of lymphoid infiltrate helps to make this distinction, which is a challenge if reviewing only core needle samples. Neuroendocrine carcinomas must have neuroendocrine morphologic features as well as neuroendocrine immunohistochemistry, findings usually absent in LECSG. Melanoma metastatic to the salivary gland is usually not cohesive, may contain pigment, and is reactive with various melanocytic markers.[131–136]

TREATMENT AND PROGNOSIS

The optimal management of LEC of the major salivary glands is complete excision with clear surgical margins followed by adjuvant radiotherapy to the tumor bed and neck. Importantly, before therapy is started, exclusion of a nasopharynx primary must be done, otherwise the field for radiotherapy may be underestimated or

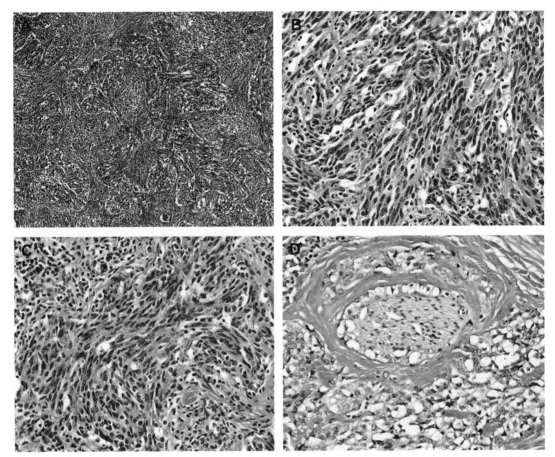

Fig. 10. (*A*) Spindled morphology with a background stroma. (*B*) Spindled morphology with histiocytes. (*C*) Spindled appearance with stippled nuclear chromatin. (*D*) Perineural invasion is easily identified.

incorrect. Several series showed that wider surgical excisions decreased the progression-free survival, and neck fibrosis was seen in patients treated with radical neck dissection, suggesting that aggressive and extended resections do not aid in tumor control or improved patient outcome.[16,34,47,121]

At the time of presentation, about 17% of patients have cervical lymph node metastases (see **Table 1**).[6,12,13,21,24,33,34,38,60,69,74,88,129,137–144] The intra–salivary gland lymph nodes are affected primarily (peripheral lymph node metastasis or by direct invasion from adjacent salivary gland), followed by the upper cervical lymph node chains, and then other lymphatic drainage basins of the neck, including the supraclavicular nodes. Imaging findings during work-up, especially to exclude a nasopharyngeal primary, usually highlight abnormal lymph nodes. Although personalized to the individual patient and local practices, elective neck dissections are not usually indicated, reserved for biopsy-proven metastases or

suspicious findings on imaging.[6,21,34,60,88] Lymph node status at presentation, extra–salivary gland extension, and marginal status do not seem to affect prognosis.[47,49] Although radiation is generally used after surgery, combination surgery and radiation therapy is only documented in 156 of 438 patients reported in the literature (see **Table 1**). It may be that therapy was excluded from the article, data was aggregated, or the treatment and outcome were not the end points of the evaluation. Suffice it to say that large clinicopathologic series included radiation in the management,[4,6,12,20,21,24,26,32,37,38,49,60,74,82,88] and it is well known that LEC is highly radiosensitive with high rates of locoregional tumor control. However, additional study is needed to establish the appropriate radiation field and dose for LECSG.[35] It has been suggested that submandibular gland tumors tend to present at higher stages and are associated with worse outcome,[47] but, when the aggregated literature is reviewed, only 3 of 36 reported patients had developed local or

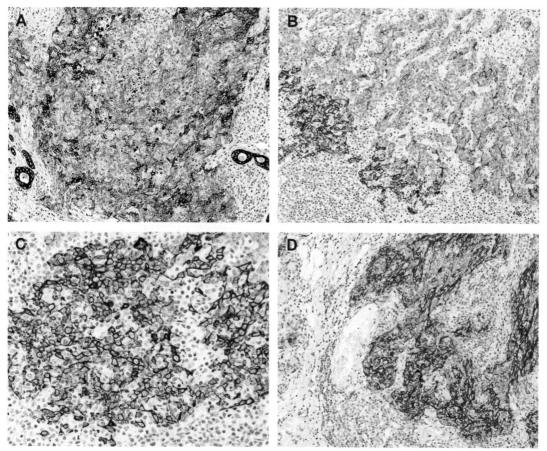

Fig. 11. Variable reactivity in the neoplastic cells with: (*A*) pancytokeratin in a solid to latticelike reaction; (*B*) reactivity with AE1/AE3 shows a strong to more patchy reactivity; (*C*) diffuse cytoplasmic reaction with keratin; (*D*) CK5/6 shows a strong membranous reactivity.

metastatic disease, and 2 had died with disease (6%), which is lower than the 26 of 141 who had died of disease overall (18.4%). Overall, 26 of 438 patients developed distant metastasis (5.9%), which was strongly correlated with death caused by the disease (69%).[2,6,24,32,34,38,47,49,60,69,88,129,145] This trend was observed more in patients from endemic areas than in those from nonendemic areas.[47] When distant metastases are identified, they are most common to lung, bones, liver, kidney, brain, spleen, and mediastinum.

When aggregating the literature (follow-up available in 141 patients), 114 of 141 patients were alive (mean follow-up of 60.7 months), whereas 22 of 141 were dead with disease (mean follow-up, 46.2 months), suggesting an overall 81% 5-year raw survival (see **Table 1**).[16,34,44,47,60,66,73,137,146] Therefore, it seems that lymph node metastases do not alter outcome, with a generally excellent

response of this tumor type to radiotherapy. The tumor category has a better prognosis than other undifferentiated carcinomas of the salivary gland (such as neuroendocrine carcinoma, NUT carcinoma, metastatic SCC), and thus correct classification is warranted in order to appropriately treat these uncommon neoplasms.

SUMMARY

Irrespective of race or ethnicity, LECSG may express EBER and is sensitive to radiation. Concurrent lymphoepithelial lesions may help suggest a primary tumor; even so, it cannot be emphasized enough that a clinical evaluation for an alternative primary should be performed. There is overall good survival, especially because of tumor radiosensitivity.

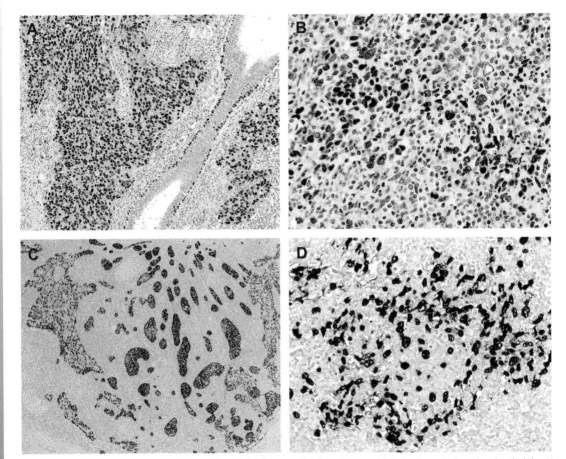

Fig. 12. (*A*) There is a strong reactivity with p63 in the neoplastic cells (basal internal control in the duct). (*B*) p40 highlights the individual neoplastic cells within the background lymphoid stroma. (*C*) Two patterns of reactivity with EBER in situ hybridization (ISH), highlighting the 2 major patterns of growth. (*D*) Single, atypical neoplastic cells show strong EBER-ISH reactivity.

CLINICS CARE POINTS

- Exclusion of a primary tumor outside of the salivary gland is paramount. These tumors are sensitive to radiation but the primary must be included in the field of treatment.

- Concurrent lymphoepithelial lesions may help suggest a primary tumor; even so, it cannot be emphasized enough that a clinical evaluation for an alternative primary should be performed.

Pitfall

! Morphology, immunohistochemical stains, and EBER-ISH are insufficient to distinguish lymphoepithelial carcinoma from nasopharyngeal carcinoma, which requires clinical evaluation.

DISCLOSURE

Both authors declare that they have no conflict of interest related to this research project. The opinions or assertions contained herein are the private views of the authors and are not to be construed as official or as reflecting the views of Southern California Permanente Medical Group.

REFERENCES

1. Lewis JS, El-Mofty SK, Nicolai P. Lymphoepithelial Carcinoma. In: El-Naggar AK, Chan JKC, Grandis JR, et al, editors. WHO classification of head and neck tumors. Lyon (France): IARC; 2017. p. 181–2.
2. Hilderman WC, Gordon JS, Large HL Jr, et al. Malignant lymphoepithelial lesion with carcinomatous component apparently arising in parotid gland. A malignant counterpart of benign lymphoepithelial lesion? Cancer 1962;15:606–10.

3. Batsakis JG. Pathology consultation. Carcinoma ex lymphoepithelial lesion. Ann Otol Rhinol Laryngol 1983;92:657–8.

4. Hamilton-Dutoit SJ, Therkildsen MH, Neilsen NH, et al. Undifferentiated carcinoma of the salivary gland in Greenlandic Eskimos: demonstration of Epstein-Barr virus DNA by in situ nucleic acid hybridization. Hum Pathol 1991;22:811–5.

5. Kuo T, Hsueh C. Lymphoepithelioma-like salivary gland carcinoma in Taiwan: a clinicopathological study of nine cases demonstrating a strong association with Epstein-Barr virus. Histopathology 1997;31:75–82.

6. Leung SY, Chung LP, Yuen ST, et al. Lymphoepithelial carcinoma of the salivary gland: in situ detection of Epstein-Barr virus. J Clin Pathol 1995;48:1022–7.

7. Manoukian JJ, Attia EL, Baxter JD, et al. Undifferentiated carcinoma with lymphoid stroma of the parotid gland. J Otolaryngol 1984;13:147–52.

8. Cleary KR, Batsakis JG. Undifferentiated carcinoma with lymphoid stroma of the major salivary glands. Ann Otol Rhinol Laryngol 1990;99:236–8.

9. Arthaud JB. Anaplastic parotid carcinoma ("malignant lymphoepithelial lesion") in seven Alaskan natives. Am J Clin Pathol 1972;57:275–86.

10. Ferlito A, Donati LF. Malignant lymphoepithelial lesions' (undifferentiated ductal carcinomas of the parotid gland). Three case reports and review of the literature. J Laryngol Otol 1977;91:869–83.

11. Nielsen NH, Mikkelsen F, Hansen JP. Incidence of salivary gland neoplasms in Greenland with special reference to an anaplastic carcinoma. Acta Pathol Microbiol Scand A 1978;86:185–93.

12. Hanji D, Gohao L. Malignant lymphoepithelial lesions of the salivary glands with anaplastic carcinomatous change. Report of nine cases and review of literature. Cancer 1983;52:2245–52.

13. Amaral AL, Nascimento AG. Malignant lymphoepithelial lesion of the submandibular gland. Oral Surg Oral Med Oral Pathol 1984;58:184–90.

14. Thompson LD. Update on nasopharyngeal carcinoma. Head Neck Pathol 2007;1:81–6.

15. Thompson LDR. Head and Neck Cancer. In: Stewart BW, Wild CP, editors. World cancer report. Lyon (France): IARCPress; 2014. p. 422–35.

16. Wenig BM. Lymphoepithelial-like carcinomas of the head and neck. Semin Diagn Pathol 2015;32:74–86.

17. Boysen T, Friborg J, Andersen A, et al. The Inuit cancer pattern–the influence of migration. Int J Cancer 2008;122:2568–72.

18. Lung ML, Chang GC, Miller TR, et al. Genotypic analysis of Epstein-Barr virus isolates associated with nasopharyngeal carcinoma in Chinese immigrants to the United States. Int J Cancer 1994;59:743–6.

19. Steinitz R, Iscovich JM, Katz L. Cancer incidence in young offspring of Jewish immigrants to Israel. A methodological study. I. Nasopharyngeal malignancies and Ewing sarcoma. Cancer Detect Prev 1990;14:547–53.

20. Saku T, Cheng J, Jen KY, et al. Epstein-Barr virus infected lymphoepithelial carcinomas of the salivary gland in the Russia-Asia area: a clinicopathologic study of 160 cases. Arkh Patol 2003;65:35–9.

21. Tsai CC, Chen CL, Hsu HC. Expression of Epstein-Barr virus in carcinomas of major salivary glands: a strong association with lymphoepithelioma-like carcinoma. Hum Pathol 1996;27:258–62.

22. Albeck H, Nielsen NH, Hansen HE, et al. Epidemiology of nasopharyngeal and salivary gland carcinoma in Greenland. Arctic Med Res 1992;51:189–95.

23. Krishnamurthy S, Lanier AP, Dohan P, et al. Salivary gland cancer in Alaskan natives, 1966-1980. Hum Pathol 1987;18:986–96.

24. Wallace AC, MacDougall JT, Hildes JA, et al. Salivary gland tumors in Canadian Eskimos. Cancer 1963;16:1338–53.

25. Bialas M, Sinczak A, Choinska-Stefanska A, et al. EBV-positive lymphoepithelial carcinoma of salivary gland in a woman of a non-endemic area–a case report. Pol J Pathol 2002;53:235–8.

26. Chan JK, Yip TT, Tsang WY, et al. Specific association of Epstein-Barr virus with lymphoepithelial carcinoma among tumors and tumorlike lesions of the salivary gland. Arch Pathol Lab Med 1994;118:994–7.

27. Dundar A, Derekoy S, Onder T, et al. Undifferentiated carcinoma with lymphoid stroma of the parotid gland. J Laryngol Otol 1993;107:1177–9.

28. Gallo O, Santucci M, Calzolari A, et al. Epstein-Barr virus (EBV) infection and undifferentiated carcinoma of the parotid gland in Caucasian patients. Acta Otolaryngol 1994;114:572–5.

29. Hamilton-Dutoit SJ, Pallesen G. Detection of Epstein-Barr virus small RNAs in routine paraffin sections using non-isotopic RNA/RNA in situ hybridization. Histopathology 1994;25:101–11.

30. Kotsianti A, Costopoulos J, Morgello S, et al. Undifferentiated carcinoma of the parotid gland in a white patient: detection of Epstein-Barr virus by in situ hybridization. Hum Pathol 1996;27:87–90.

31. Kott ET, Goepfert H, Ayala AG, et al. Lymphoepithelial carcinoma (malignant lymphoepithelial lesion) of the salivary glands. Arch Otolaryngol 1984;110:50–3.

32. Lanier AP, Clift SR, Bornkamm G, et al. Epstein-Barr virus and malignant lymphoepithelial lesions of the salivary gland. Arctic Med Res 1991;50:55–61.

33. Larbcharoensub N, Tubtong N, Praneetvatakul V, et al. Epstein-Barr virus associated lymphoepithelial carcinoma of the parotid gland; a

clinicopathological report of three cases. J Med Assoc Thai 2006;89:1536–41.

34. Li F, Zhu G, Wang Y, et al. A clinical analysis of 37 cases with lymphoepithelial carcinoma of the major salivary gland treated by surgical resection and postoperative radiotherapy: a single institution study. Med Oncol 2014;31:957.

35. Manganaris A, Patakiouta F, Xirou P, et al. Lymphoepithelial carcinoma of the parotid gland: is an association with Epstein-Barr virus possible in non-endemic areas? Int J Oral Maxillofac Surg 2007;36:556–9.

36. Mrad K, Ben Brahim E, Driss M, et al. Lymphoepithelioma-like carcinoma of the submandibular salivary gland associated with Epstein-Barr virus in a North African woman. Virchows Arch 2004;445: 419–20.

37. Nagao T, Ishida Y, Sugano I, et al. Epstein-Barr virus-associated undifferentiated carcinoma with lymphoid stroma of the salivary gland in Japanese patients. Comparison with benign lymphoepithelial lesion. Cancer 1996;78:695–703.

38. Bosch JD, Kudryk WH, Johnson GH. The malignant lymphoepithelial lesion of the salivary glands. J Otolaryngol 1988;17:187–90.

39. Chen KT. Carcinoma arising in a benign lymphoepithelial lesion. Arch Otolaryngol 1983;109: 619–21.

40. Christiansen MS, Mourad WA, Hales ML, et al. Spindle cell malignant lymphoepithelial lesion of the parotid gland: clinical, light microscopic, ultrastructural, and in situ hybridization findings in one case. Mod Pathol 1995;8:711–5.

41. Falzon M, Isaacson PG. The natural history of benign lymphoepithelial lesion of the salivary gland in which there is a monoclonal population of B cells. A report of two cases. Am J Surg Pathol 1991;15: 59–65.

42. Gleeson MJ, Cawson RA, Bennett MH. Benign lymphoepithelial lesion: a less than benign disease. Clin Otolaryngol Allied Sci 1986;11:47–51.

43. Kitazawa M, Ohnishi Y, Nonomura N, et al. Malignant lymphoepithelial lesion. Acta Pathol Jpn 1987;37:515–26.

44. Ma Q, Song H. Diagnosis and management of lymphoepithelial lesion of the parotid gland. Rheumatol Int 2011;31:959–62.

45. Nagao K, Matsuzaki O, Saiga H, et al. A histopathologic study of benign and malignant lymphoepithelial lesions of the parotid gland. Cancer 1983;52:1044–52.

46. Schneider M, Rizzardi C. Lymphoepithelial carcinoma of the parotid glands and its relationship with benign lymphoepithelial lesions. Arch Pathol Lab Med 2008;132:278–82.

47. Zhan KY, Nicolli EA, Khaja SF, et al. Lymphoepithelial carcinoma of the major salivary glands: Predictors of survival in a non-endemic region. Oral Oncol 2016;52:24–9.

48. Mozaffari HR, Ramezani M, Janbakhsh A, et al. Malignant Salivary Gland Tumors and Epstein-Barr virus (EBV) Infection: A Systematic Review and Meta-Analysis. Asian Pac J Cancer Prev 2017;18: 1201–6.

49. Whaley RD, Carlos R, Bishop JA, et al. Lymphoepithelial carcinoma of salivary gland EBV-association in endemic versus non-endemic patients: A report of 16 cases. Head Neck Pathol 2020. https://doi.org/10.1007/s12105-020-01172-w.

50. Weiss LM, Gaffey MJ, Shibata D. Lymphoepithelioma-like carcinoma and its relationship to Epstein-Barr virus. Am J Clin Pathol 1991;96:156–8.

51. Pittaluga S, Wong MP, Chung LP, et al. Clonal Epstein-Barr virus in lymphoepithelioma-like carcinoma of the lung. Am J Surg Pathol 1993;17:678–82.

52. Wang D, Liebowitz D, Kieff E. An EBV membrane protein expressed in immortalized lymphocytes transforms established rodent cells. Cell 1985;43:831–40.

53. Henderson S, Rowe M, Gregory C, et al. Induction of bcl-2 expression by Epstein-Barr virus latent membrane protein 1 protects infected B cells from programmed cell death. Cell 1991;65:1107–15.

54. Dawson CW, Rickinson AB, Young LS. Epstein-Barr virus latent membrane protein inhibits human epithelial cell differentiation. Nature 1990;344: 777–80.

55. Shebl FM, Bhatia K, Engels EA. Salivary gland and nasopharyngeal cancers in individuals with acquired immunodeficiency syndrome in United States. Int J Cancer 2010;126:2503–8.

56. Ellis GL. Lymphoid lesions of salivary glands: malignant and benign. Med Oral Patol Oral Cir Bucal 2007;12:E479–85.

57. Maiorano E, Favia G, Viale G. Lymphoepithelial cysts of salivary glands: an immunohistochemical study of HIV-related and HIV-unrelated lesions. Hum Pathol 1998;29:260–5.

58. Sujatha D, Babitha K, Prasad RS, et al. Parotid lymphoepithelial cysts in human immunodeficiency virus: a review. J Laryngol Otol 2013;127:1046–9.

59. Wu L, Cheng J, Maruyama S, et al. Lymphoepithelial cyst of the parotid gland: its possible histopathogenesis based on clinicopathologic analysis of 64 cases. Hum Pathol 2009;40:683–92.

60. Wang CP, Chang YL, Ko JY, et al. Lymphoepithelial carcinoma versus large cell undifferentiated carcinoma of the major salivary glands. Cancer 2004; 101:2020–7.

61. Zhang Q, Qing J, Wei MW, et al. [Clinical analysis of sixteen cases of lymphoepithelial carcinoma of salivary gland]. Ai Zheng 2005;24:1384–7.

62. Li LJ, Li Y, Wen YM, et al. Clinical analysis of salivary gland tumor cases in West China in past 50 years. Oral Oncol 2008;44:187–92.

63. Tian Z, Li L, Wang L, et al. Salivary gland neo-plasms in oral and maxillofacial regions: a 23-year retrospective study of 6982 cases in an eastern Chinese population. Int J Oral Maxillofac Surg 2010;39:235–42.

64. Wang YL, Zhu YX, Chen TZ, et al. Clinicopathologic study of 1176 salivary gland tumors in a Chinese population: experience of one cancer center 1997-2007. Acta Otolaryngol 2012;132:879–86.

65. Jones AV, Craig GT, Speight PM, et al. The range and demographics of salivary gland tumours diagnosed in a UK population. Oral Oncol 2008;44:407–17.

66. Sheen TS, Tsai CC, Ko JY, et al. Undifferentiated carcinoma of the major salivary glands. Cancer 1997;80:357–63.

67. Abdelkrim SB, Trabelsi A, Hammedi F, et al. Primary lymphoepithelial carcinoma of the parotid gland in a North African woman. Rare Tumors 2009;1:e16.

68. Autio-Harmainen H, Paakko P, Alavaikko M, et al. Familial occurrence of malignant lymphoepithelial lesion of the parotid gland in a Finnish family with dominantly inherited trichoepithelioma. Cancer 1988;61:161–6.

69. Saqui-Salces M, Martinez-Benitez B, Gamboa-Dominguez A. EBV+ lymphoepithelial carcinoma of the parotid gland in Mexican Mestizo patients with chronic autoimmune diseases. Pathol Oncol Res 2006;12:41–5.

70. Ban X, Wu J, Mo Y, et al. Lymphoepithelial carcinoma of the salivary gland: morphologic patterns and imaging features on CT and MRI. AJNR Am J Neuroradiol 2014;35:1813–9.

71. Wang P, Yang J, Yu Q. Lymphoepithelial carcinoma of salivary glands: CT and MR imaging findings. Dentomaxillofac Radiol 2017;46:20170053.

72. Yao L, Zhang Y, Chen Q, et al. Diagnosis of lymphoepithelial carcinoma in parotid gland with three dimensional computed tomography angiography reconstruction: A case report. J Xray Sci Technol 2018;26:155–64.

73. Zhang G, Tang J, Pan Y, et al. CT features and pathologic characteristics of lymphoepithelial carcinoma of salivary glands. Int J Clin Exp Pathol 2014;7:1004–11.

74. Saw D, Lau WH, Ho JH, et al. Malignant lymphoepithelial lesion of the salivary gland. Hum Pathol 1986;17:914–23.

75. Gunhan O, Celasun B, Safali M, et al. Fine needle aspiration cytology of malignant lymphoepithelial lesion of the salivary gland. A report of two cases. Acta Cytol 1994;38:751–4.

76. Safneck JR, Ravinsky E, Yazdi HM, et al. Fine needle aspiration biopsy findings in lymphoepithelial carcinoma of salivary gland. Acta Cytol 1997;41:1023–30.

77. Yazdi HM, Hogg GR. Malignant lymphoepithelial lesion of the submandibular salivary gland. Am J Clin Pathol 1984;82:344–8.

78. Hipp JA, Jing X, Zarka MA, et al. Cytomorphologic characteristics and differential diagnoses of lymphoepithelial carcinoma of the parotid. J Am Soc Cytopathol 2016;5:93–9.

79. Kim KI, Kim YS, Kim HK, et al. The detection of Epstein-Barr virus in the lesions of salivary glands. Pathol Res Pract 1999;195:407–12.

80. James PD, Ellis IO. Malignant epithelial tumours associated with autoimmune sialadenitis. J Clin Pathol 1986;39:497–502.

81. DiGiuseppe JA, Corio RL, Westra WH. Lymphoid infiltrates of the salivary glands: pathology, biology and clinical significance. Curr Opin Oncol 1996;8:232–7.

82. Friborg J, Hamilton-Therkildsen M, Homoe P, et al. A spectrum of basaloid morphology in a subset of EBV-associated "lymphoepithelial carcinomas" of major salivary glands. Head Neck Pathol 2012;6:445–50.

83. Kurian EM, Miller R, McLean-Holden AL, et al. Low Molecular Weight Cytokeratin Immunostaining for Extrafollicular Reticulum Cells is an Effective Means of Separating Salivary Gland Tumor-Associated Lymphoid Proliferation from True Lymph Node Involvement. Head Neck Pathol 2019;14(3):593–7.

84. Herbst H, Niedobitek G. Sporadic EBV-associated lymphoepithelial salivary gland carcinoma with EBV-positive low-grade myoepithelial component. Virchows Arch 2006;448:648–54.

85. Redondo C, Garcia A, Vazquez F. Malignant lymphoepithelial lesion of the parotid gland: poorly differentiated squamous cell carcinoma with lymphoid stroma. Cancer 1981;48:289–92.

86. Sehested M, Hainau B, Albeck H, et al. Ultrastructural investigation of anaplastic salivary gland carcinomas in Eskimos. Cancer 1985;55:2732–6.

87. Lu SY, Huang CC, Hsiung CY, et al. Primary lymphoepithelioma-like carcinoma of minor salivary gland: a case report with immunohistochemical and in situ hybridization studies. Head Neck 2006;28:182–6.

88. Zhao W, Deng N, Gao X, et al. Primary lymphoepithelioma-like carcinoma of salivary glands: a clinicopathological study of 21 cases. Int J Clin Exp Pathol 2014;7:7951–6.

89. Rooper LM, McCuiston AM, Westra WH, et al. SOX10 Immunoexpression in Basaloid Squamous Cell Carcinomas: A Diagnostic Pitfall for Ruling out Salivary Differentiation. Head Neck Pathol 2018;13(4):543–7.

90. Jen KY, Cheng J, Li J, et al. Mutational events in LMP1 gene of Epstein-Barr virus in salivary gland lymphoepithelial carcinomas. Int J Cancer 2003;105:654–60.

91. Cruickshank AH. Benign lymphoepithelial salivary lesion to be distinguished from adenolymphoma. J Clin Pathol 1965;18:391–400.

92. Geyer JT, Ferry JA, Harris NL, et al. Chronic sclerosing sialadenitis (Kuttner tumor) is an IgG4-associated disease. Am J Surg Pathol 2010;34:202–10.

93. Andreasen S, Varma S, Barasch N, et al. The HTN3-MSANTD3 Fusion Gene Defines a Subset of Acinic Cell Carcinoma of the Salivary Gland. Am J Surg Pathol 2019;43:489–96.

94. Thompson LD. Salivary gland acinic cell carcinoma. Ear Nose Throat J 2010;89:530–2.

95. Thompson LD, Aslam MN, Stall JN, et al. Clinicopathologic and Immunophenotypic Characterization of 25 Cases of Acinic Cell Carcinoma with High-Grade Transformation. Head Neck Pathol 2016;10:152–60.

96. Vander Poorten V, Triantafyllou A, Thompson LD, et al. Salivary acinic cell carcinoma: reappraisal and update. Eur Arch Otorhinolaryngol 2016;273:3511–31.

97. Haller F, Bieg M, Will R, et al. Enhancer hijacking activates oncogenic transcription factor NR4A3 in acinic cell carcinomas of the salivary glands. Nat Commun 2019;10:368.

98. Tirado Y, Williams MD, Hanna EY, et al. CRTC1/MAML2 fusion transcript in high grade mucoepidermoid carcinomas of salivary and thyroid glands and Warthin's tumors: implications for histogenesis and biologic behavior. Genes Chromosomes Cancer 2007;46:708–15.

99. Nakayama T, Miyabe S, Okabe M, et al. Clinicopathological significance of the CRTC3-MAML2 fusion transcript in mucoepidermoid carcinoma. Mod Pathol 2009;22:1575–81.

100. Seethala RR, Chiosea SI. MAML2 Status in Mucoepidermoid Carcinoma Can No Longer Be Considered a Prognostic Marker. Am J Surg Pathol 2016;40:1151–3.

101. Bishop JA, Cowan ML, Shum CH, et al. MAML2 Rearrangements in Variant Forms of Mucoepidermoid Carcinoma: Ancillary Diagnostic Testing for the Ciliated and Warthin-like Variants. Am J Surg Pathol 2018;42:130–6.

102. Skalova A, Stenman G, Simpson RHW, et al. The Role of Molecular Testing in the Differential Diagnosis of Salivary Gland Carcinomas. Am J Surg Pathol 2018;42:e11–27.

103. Prasad ML, Chiosea S, Ihrler S, et al. Tumours of salivary glands: Benign neoplasms: Lymphadenoma. In: El-Naggar AK, Chan JKC, Grandis JR, et al, editors. WHO classification of head and neck tumours. Lyon (France): IARC; 2017. p. 190–1.

104. Liu G, He J, Zhang C, et al. Lymphadenoma of the salivary gland: Report of 10 cases. Oncol Lett 2014;7:1097–101.

105. Seethala RR, Thompson LD, Gnepp DR, et al. Lymphadenoma of the salivary gland: clinicopathological and immunohistochemical analysis of 33 tumors. Mod Pathol 2012;25:26–35.

106. Patel DK, Morton RP. Demographics of benign parotid tumours: Warthin's tumour versus other benign salivary tumours. Acta Otolaryngol 2016;136:83–6.

107. Schmitt AC, Cohen C, Siddiqui MT. Expression of SOX10 in Salivary Gland Oncocytic Neoplasms: A Review and a Comparative Analysis with Other Immunohistochemical Markers. Acta Cytol 2015;59:384–90.

108. Chedid HM, Rapoport A, Aikawa KF, et al. Warthin's tumor of the parotid gland: study of 70 cases. Rev Col Bras Cir 2011;38:90–4.

109. Chu CY, Pan SC, Chang KC. EBV-positive diffuse large B-cell lymphoma of the elderly involving Warthin tumor. Pathol Int 2015;65:677–9.

110. van Heerden WF, Kraft K, Hemmer J, et al. Warthin's tumour is not an Epstein-Barr virus related disease. Anticancer Res 1999;19:2881–3.

111. Ozkok G, Tasli F, Ozsan N, et al. Diffuse Large B-Cell Lymphoma Arising in Warthin's Tumor: Case Study and Review of the Literature. Korean J Pathol 2013;47:579–82.

112. Vazquez A, Khan MN, Sanghvi S, et al. Extranodal marginal zone lymphoma of mucosa-associated lymphoid tissue of the salivary glands: a population-based study from 1994 to 2009. Head Neck 2015;37:18–22.

113. Agaimy A, Wild V, Markl B, et al. Intraparotid classical and nodular lymphocyte-predominant Hodgkin lymphoma: pattern analysis with emphasis on associated lymphadenoma-like proliferations. Am J Surg Pathol 2015;39:1206–12.

114. Mian M, Capello D, Ventre MB, et al. Early-stage diffuse large B cell lymphoma of the head and neck: clinico-biological characterization and 18 year follow-up of 488 patients (IELSG 23 study). Ann Hematol 2014;93:221–31.

115. Laviv A, Sohani AR, Troulis MJ. Lymphoma mimics obstructive sialadenitis: three cases. J Oral Maxillofac Surg 2014;72:1325.e1-11.

116. Feinstein AJ, Ciarleglio MM, Cong X, et al. Parotid gland lymphoma: prognostic analysis of 2140 patients. Laryngoscope 2013;123:1199–203.

117. Suh C, Huh J, Roh JL. Extranodal marginal zone B-cell lymphoma of mucosa-associated lymphoid tissue arising in the extracranial head and neck region: a high rate of dissemination and disease recurrence. Oral Oncol 2008;44:949–55.

118. Harris NL. Lymphoid proliferations of the salivary glands. Am J Clin Pathol 1999;111:S94–103.

119. Roh JL, Huh J, Suh C. Primary non-Hodgkin's lymphomas of the major salivary glands. J Surg Oncol 2008;97:35–9.

120. Tiplady CW, Taylor PR, White J, et al. Lymphoma presenting as a parotid tumour: a population-based study of diagnosis, treatment and outcome on behalf of the Scotland and Newcastle Lymphoma Group. Clin Oncol (R Coll Radiol) 2004; 16:414–9.

121. Kim YJ, Hong HS, Jeong SH, et al. Lymphoepithelial carcinoma of the salivary glands. Medicine (Baltimore) 2017;96:e6115.

122. Thompson LDR, Burchette R, Iganej S, et al. Oropharyngeal Squamous Cell Carcinoma in 390 Patients: Analysis of Clinical and Histological Criteria Which Significantly Impact Outcome. Head Neck Pathol 2019;14(3):666–88.

123. Carpenter DH, El-Mofty SK, Lewis JS Jr. Undifferentiated carcinoma of the oropharynx: a human papillomavirus-associated tumor with a favorable prognosis. Mod Pathol 2011;24:1306–12.

124. Singhi AD, Stelow EB, Mills SE, et al. Lymphoepithelial-like carcinoma of the oropharynx: a morphologic variant of HPV-related head and neck carcinoma. Am J Surg Pathol 2010;34:800–5.

125. Agaimy A, Fonseca I, Martins C, et al. NUT Carcinoma of the Salivary Glands: Clinicopathologic and Molecular Analysis of 3 Cases and a Survey of NUT Expression in Salivary Gland Carcinomas. Am J Surg Pathol 2018;42:877–84.

126. Rooper LM, Jo VY, Antonescu CR, et al. Adamantinoma-like Ewing Sarcoma of the Salivary Glands: A Newly Recognized Mimicker of Basaloid Salivary Carcinomas. Am J Surg Pathol 2019;43:187–94.

127. Lilo MT, Bishop JA, Olson MT, et al. Adamantinoma-like Ewing sarcoma of the parotid gland: Cytopathologic findings and differential diagnosis. Diagn Cytopathol 2018;46:263–6.

128. Batsakis JG, Luna MA. Undifferentiated carcinomas of salivary glands. Ann Otol Rhinol Laryngol 1991;100:82–4.

129. Hatta C, Terada T, Okita J, et al. Clinicopathological study of undifferentiated carcinoma of the parotid gland. Auris Nasus Larynx 2003;30:273–7.

130. Hui KK, Luna MA, Batsakis JG, et al. Undifferentiated carcinomas of the major salivary glands. Oral Surg Oral Med Oral Pathol 1990;69:76–83.

131. Wick MR. Primary lesions that may imitate metastatic tumors histologically: A selective review. Semin Diagn Pathol 2018;35:123–42.

132. Bron LP, Traynor SJ, McNeil EB, et al. Primary and metastatic cancer of the parotid: comparison of clinical behavior in 232 cases. Laryngoscope 2003;113:1070–5.

133. Den Hondt M, Starr MW, Millett MC, et al. Surgical management of the neck in patients with metastatic melanoma in parotid lymph nodes. J Surg Oncol 2019;120:1462–9.

134. Wang H, Hoda RS, Faquin W, et al. FNA biopsy of secondary nonlymphomatous malignancies in salivary glands: A multi-institutional study of 184 cases. Cancer Cytopathol 2017;125:91–103.

135. Pastore A, Ciorba A, Soliani M, et al. Secondary malignant tumors of the parotid gland: not a secondary problem! J Buon 2017;22:513–8.

136. Thom JJ, Moore EJ, Price DL, et al. The Role of Total Parotidectomy for Metastatic Cutaneous Squamous Cell Carcinoma and Malignant Melanoma. JAMA Otolaryngol Head Neck Surg 2014;140:548–54.

137. Abdulla AK, Mian MY. Lymphoepithelial carcinoma of salivary glands. Head Neck 1996;18:577–81.

138. Delaney WE, Balogh K Jr. Carcinoma of the parotid gland associated with benign lymphoepithelial lesion (Mikulicz's disease) in Sjogren's syndrome. Cancer 1966;19:853–60.

139. Sinha BK, Buntine DW. Parotid gland tumors. Clinicopathologic study. Am J Surg 1975;129:675–81.

140. Batsakis JG, Bernacki EG, Rice DH, et al. Malignancy and the benign lymphoepithelial lesion. Laryngoscope 1975;85:389–99.

141. Gravanis MB, Giansanti JS. Malignant histopathologic counterpart of the benign lymphoepithelial lesion. Cancer 1970;26:1332–42.

142. Jang SJ, Paik SS, Lee WM, et al. Lymphoepithelial carcinoma of the submandibular gland–a case report. J Korean Med Sci 1997;12:252–5.

143. Kountakis SE, SooHoo W, Maillard A. Lymphoepithelial carcinoma of the parotid gland. Head Neck 1995;17:445–50.

144. Worley NK, Daroca PJ Jr. Lymphoepithelial carcinoma of the minor salivary gland. Arch Otolaryngol Head Neck Surg 1997;123:638–40.

145. Batsakis JG. The pathology of head and neck tumors: the lymphoepithelial lesion and Sjogren's syndrome, Part 16. Head Neck Surg 1982;5:150–63.

146. Hsiung CY, Huang CC, Wang CJ, et al. Lymphoepithelioma-like carcinoma of salivary glands: treatment results and failure patterns. Br J Radiol 2006;79:52–5.

147. Borg MF, Benjamin CS, Morton RP, et al. Malignant lympho-epithelial lesion of the salivary gland: a case report and review of the literature. Australas Radiol 1993;37:288–91.

148. Gokdogan O, Koybasioglu A. Recurrent Lymphoepithelial Carcinoma of the Parotid Gland. J Craniofac Surg 2015;26:e543–5.

149. Halder A, Sommerville J, Gandhi M. Primary lymphoepthelial carcinoma of the parotid gland, pictorial review of a rare entity. J Med Imaging Radiat Oncol 2018;62:355–60.

150. Jayaram G, Peh SC. Lymphoepithelial carcinoma of salivary gland - cytologic, histologic, immunocytochemical, and in situ hybridization features in a case. Diagn Cytopathol 2000;22:400–2.

151. Maeda H, Yamashiro T, Yamashita Y, et al. Lymphoepithelial carcinoma in parotid gland related to EBV infection: A case report. Auris Nasus Larynx 2018;45:170–4.

152. Menditti D, Laino L, Milano M, et al. Intraoral lymphoepithelial carcinoma of the minor salivary glands. In Vivo 2012;26:1087–9.

153. Merrick Y, Albeck H, Nielsen NH, et al. Familial clustering of salivary gland carcinoma in Greenland. Cancer 1986;57:2097–102.

154. Roncevic R, Tatic V. Malignant lymphoepithelial lesion: report of case. J Oral Surg 1981;39:449–50.

155. Roy L, Moubayed SP, Ayad T. Lymphoepithelial Carcinoma of the Sublingual Gland: Case Report and Review of the Literature. J Oral Maxillofac Surg 2015;73:1878.e1-5.

156. Stanley MW, Bardales RH, Farmer CE, et al. Primary and metastatic high-grade carcinomas of the salivary glands: a cytologic-histologic correlation study of twenty cases. Diagn Cytopathol 1995;13:37–43.

157. Tang CG, Schmidtknecht TM, Tang GY, et al. Lymphoepithelial carcinoma: a case of a rare parotid gland tumor. Perm J 2012;16:60–2.

158. Topal O, Erinanc H. Coexistence of Lymphoepithelial Carcinoma of the Parotid Gland and Submandibular Gland Pleomorphic Adenoma. J Craniofac Surg 2017;28:e453–4.

159. Wu DL, Shemen L, Brady T, et al. Malignant lymphoepithelial lesion of the parotid gland: a case report and review of the literature. Ear Nose Throat J 2001;80:803–6.

160. Zeng M, Li S, Fu J, et al. Primary lymphoepithelial carcinoma of the intraoral minor salivary gland: A case report. Oncol Lett 2015;9:790–2.

Epithelial–Myoepithelial Carcinoma

Masato Nakaguro, MD, PhD[a], Toshitaka Nagao, MD, PhD[b],*

KEYWORDS

• Epithelial-myoepithelial carcinoma • Biphasic differentiation • *HRAS* • Salivary gland tumor

Key points

- Epithelial–myoepithelial carcinoma is an uncommon low-grade salivary gland carcinoma.

- Classically, epithelial–myoepithelial carcinoma is characterized by biphasic tubular structures composed of inner eosinophilic ductal cells and outer clear myoepithelial cells.

- In addition to classical histology, there are several histologic variations in epithelial–myoepithelial carcinoma.

- The differential diagnosis includes many other salivary gland tumor types showing biphasic differentiation as well as clear cell morphology.

- *HRAS* mutations are a frequent genetic event in and specific to epithelial–myoepithelial carcinoma.

ABSTRACT

Epithelial–myoepithelial carcinoma is an uncommon low-grade salivary gland carcinoma. It is classically characterized by biphasic tubular structures composed of inner eosinophilic ductal cells and outer clear myoepithelial cells. In addition, epithelial–myoepithelial carcinoma sometimes shows various histologic features, including a cribriform pattern, basaloid appearance, and sebaceous differentiation. Because clear myoepithelial cells are also noted in other benign and malignant salivary gland tumors, the histologic variety and similarity with other tumor entities make the diagnosis of epithelial–myoepithelial carcinoma challenging. A recent analysis revealed that *HRAS* hotspot point mutations are specifically identified in epithelial–myoepithelial carcinoma and the assessment of given genes facilitate the correct diagnosis.

OVERVIEW

Epithelial–myoepithelial carcinoma (EMC) is a low-grade and uncommon salivary gland neoplasm, accounting for 1% of all salivary gland tumors and 2% of all salivary gland malignancies.[1,2] It typically occurs in the sixth and seventh decades of life and has an even sex distribution or a slight female predilection.[3,4] EMC typically presents as a slow-growing painless mass. Facial nerve symptoms and lymphadenopathy are rare.[3] More than three-quarters of EMCs develop in the parotid gland; the remainder affect the other major or minor salivary glands, lacrimal gland, and seromucinous glands in the sinonasal tract or bronchus.[2–4] EMC is usually indolent, but local recurrence is not uncommon.[3]

The designation EMC was first introduced in 1972 by Donath and colleagues,[5] and since then many articles and textbooks have described this

[a] Department of Pathology and Laboratory Medicine, Nagoya University Hospital, 65 Tsurumai-cho, Showa-ku, Nagoya, Japan; [b] Department of Anatomic Pathology, Tokyo Medical University, 6-7-1 Nishishinjuku, Shinjuku-ku, Tokyo, Japan
* Corresponding author.
E-mail address: nagao-t@tokyo-med.ac.jp
Twitter: @assamusic (M.N.)

Surgical Pathology 14 (2021) 97–109
https://doi.org/10.1016/j.path.2020.10.002

entity. However, because there is some overlap of its histologic features with various other tumor types, the diagnosis of EMC remains challenging. In the *World Health Organization Classification of Head and Neck Tumors 4th Edition*,[3] EMC is defined as "a malignant salivary gland tumor composed of a biphasic arrangement of inner luminal ductal cells and outer myoepithelial cells." However, other salivary gland malignancies with biphasic differentiation, such as adenoid cystic carcinoma (AdCC) and basal cell adenocarcinoma (BCAC), also meet this criterion. Therefore, the characteristic cytologic features, namely, the presence of eosinophilic ductal cells and clear myoepithelial cells, at least those seen in a classical case, must be included in the diagnostic criteria of EMC.

In addition to the classical forms, a wide range of histologic variations can be observed in EMC. Consequently, the careful evaluation of the whole tumor, including the tumor border, and the cautious exclusion of other tumor types are required to make a correct diagnosis of EMC.

GROSS FEATURES

The reported mean tumor size is 2.9 to 3.5 cm (range, 0.5–8.0 cm).[1,4] The cut surface typically shows a white to tan, nodular, firm mass with partial encapsulation. Focal cystic changes are noted in 30% of cases.[1,3]

MICROSCOPIC FEATURES

HISTOLOGY (BOX 1)

EMC generally displays a well-circumscribed mass with multilobular or multinodular growth (**Fig. 1A**). The tumor is usually surrounded at least focally by a capsule-like fibrous tissue with minimal invasion.[1] Unlike AdCCs, frankly infiltrative lesions with an ill-defined boundary are less frequent and account for 23% of EMCs.[1] Classically, EMC is characterized by a biphasic tubular structure

of inner (luminal) eosinophilic ductal epithelial cells and outer (abluminal) clear myoepithelial cells (**Fig. 1B**).[2,3] The neoplastic tubules are frequently encased by a basement membrane-like hyaline material, that differs from myoepithelial cells blending into myxomatous elements seen in pleomorphic adenoma (PA).[6] The lumens of the tubules occasionally contain eosinophilic secretions. Although the proportion of the 2-cell type varies among cases, myoepithelial cells usually outnumber luminal ductal cells (**Fig. 1E**), and the mean myoepithelial/epithelial ratio is 1.8 to 4.3.[1,4] Myoepithelial cells typically show arrangement in single or multiple layers, sometimes even showing a sheet-like proliferation. Myoepithelial cells are larger than luminal ductal cells and possess round, oval, and sometimes spindle-shaped nuclei.[3] The nuclei have open chromatin and inconspicuous nucleoli. The clear cytoplasm of myoepithelial cells is caused in part by glycogen storage but largely by a tissue-processing artifact.[7] The nuclear atypia of the tumor cells is mild to moderate, and more than 90% of cases show no pleomorphism.[1,4] Mitotic figures are not prominent, and the mean mitotic counts are 3.3 to 3.6 per 10 high-power fields.[1,4] Necrosis, lymphovascular invasion, and perineural invasion have been noted in 18.0% to 19.5%, 10.3% to 11.5%, and 16.1% to 34.4% of cases, respectively.[1,4]

In addition to the classical histologic characteristics of EMC, various unusual architectural and cytologic features have been described as well.[1,4] Some have been reported as histologic variants, but according to large series studies, these histologic features are not rare and are mostly observed focally in the tumor, so they may be regarded as falling within a wide range of variation of EMC rather than being distinct variants. Among them, a cribriform pattern of growth (**Fig. 2A**), basaloid appearance (**Fig. 2B**), and sebaceous differentiation (**Fig. 2C**) are the most common (17%–18% of EMC).[4] EMC can also exhibit a papillary–cystic pattern. EMC with a

---

Box 1
Pathologic key features of EMC

- Multilobular invasive growth.

- Tubular formation consisting of Inner eosinophilic ductal epithelial cells and outer clear myoepithelial cells.

- There is overlap of its histologic features with various benign and malignant salivary gland tumors.

- Histologic variations: cribriform formation, basaloid appearance, sebaceous differentiation, apocrine/oncocytic change, papillary-cystic structure, double-clear appearance, squamous metaplasia, Verocay-like myoepithelial cells, psammomatous features, and ex pleomorphic adenoma.

- Frequent *HRAS* (Q61R) mutations.

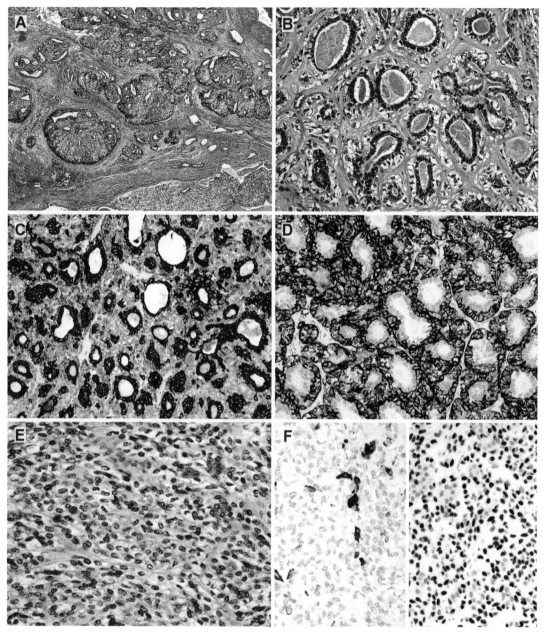

Fig. 1. Classical EMC. A low-power view shows multinodular invasive growth accompanied by intervening sclerotic stroma (*A*). Bilayered tubular structures consisting of inner eosinophilic ductal cells and outer polygonal clear myoepithelial cells (*B*). Immunohistochemically, the luminal cells and abluminal cells are strongly positive for CK7 (*C*) and α-smooth muscle actin (*D*), respectively. Clear myoepithelial cells outnumber eosinophilic ductal cells (*E*). The luminal cells are positive for pan-CK (AE1/AE3) (*F, left*) but negative for p63 (*F, right*).

prominent cribriform pattern closely resembles AdCC.[4,8,9] In contrast, basaloid EMC mimics basal cell adenoma/adenocarcinoma (BCA/BCAC).[10] Areas of sebaceous differentiation are usually present focally but occasionally seem to cover more than 50% of the tumor mass.[1,4,11] Specific myoepithelial markers are useful for differentiating EMC

from sebaceous carcinoma.[11] The oncocytic and apocrine feature (**Fig. 2D**), which is characterized by eosinophilic cytoplasm of luminal ductal cells, is also uncommonly seen in EMC (7%–8%).[1,4,12,13] It is classified as either oncocytic or apocrine in morphology and demonstrates immunohistochemical reactivity for mitochondria or androgen receptor, respectively.[12,13] EMC markedly consisting of apocrine-type cells can be distinguished from salivary duct carcinoma by the presence of myoepithelial cells.[12] EMC composed of clear luminal ductal cells and clear myoepithelial cells is referred to as double-clear EMC (**Fig. 2**E).[1,14] This unique appearance obscures its biphasic nature and can be misdiagnosed as myoepithelial carcinoma or clear cell carcinoma.[14] Squamous metaplasia (**Fig. 2**F) and Verocay-like myoepithelial cells (**Fig. 2**G) have also been described.[1,4] The presence of these findings in EMC can be difficult to distinguish from other salivary gland tumor types. Although hybrid carcinomas composed of EMC with other carcinomas, including AdCC and BCAC, have been reported,[15] most such cases should be interpreted as a histologic variation of EMC. The impact of specific histologic features on patient prognosis has not been clarified.

EMC arising in preexisting PA has been reported, but the ratio to *de novo* EMC varies markedly among studies (from 1.6% to 79.5%).[1,4,16,17]

This discrepancy may be caused by the difference in the interpretation of diagnostic criteria. However, all studies have shown that EMC ex PA cases have no or a much lower frequency of *HRAS* mutations than *de novo* EMC. For this reason, alleged EMC ex PA might actually be a distinct entity or EMC-mimicking tumor.

EMCs histologically rarely undergo high-grade transformation (**Fig. 2**H).[1] High-grade transformation is observed in 3.4% to 6.5% of EMC cases[1,4,18–22] and is defined as an abrupt transformation from original well-differentiated carcinoma into high-grade carcinoma that lacks the original distinct histologic characteristics.[22] The high-grade component, which is commonly either poorly differentiated adenocarcinoma or undifferentiated carcinoma, is characterized by pleomorphism and prominent necrosis.[22] Previously the term "dedifferentiation" was often used as a synonym, and the name myoepithelial anaplasia was also used to describe high-grade tumors with myoepithelial differentiation.[19] Because it is sometimes difficult to determine for the high-grade

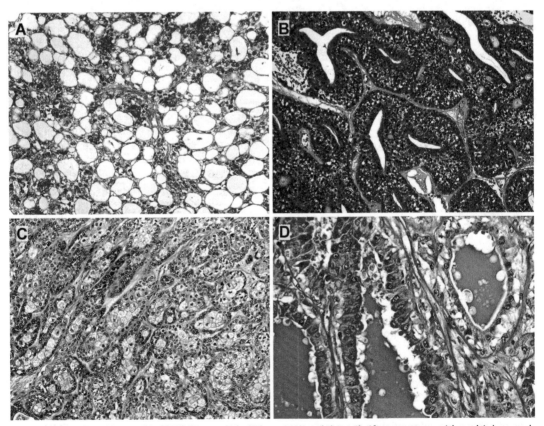

Fig. 2. Histologic variations of epithelial-myoepithelial carcinoma. (*A*) A cribriform pattern with multiple pseudocysts. (*B*) Basaloid appearance. (*C*) Sebaceous differentiation featuring tumor cells with bubbly cytoplasm. (*D*) Apocrine differentiation of ductal cells. (*E*) A double-clear tubular pattern. (*F*) Squamous differentiation. (*G*) Verocay-like myoepithelial cells. (*H*) High-grade transformation.

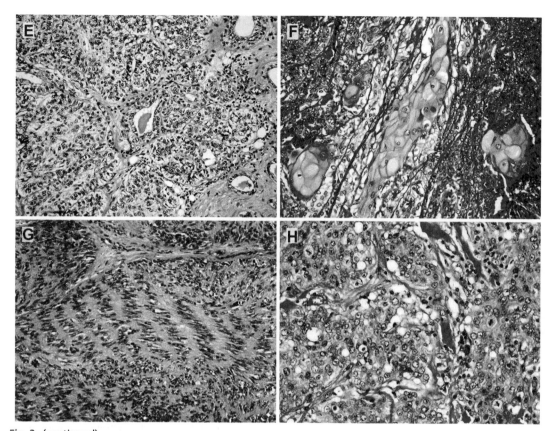

Fig. 2. (continued)

component whether it originates from luminal ductal cells or myoepithelial cells by histomorphology or immunohistochemistry, the more comprehensive designation high-grade transformation seems to be justified and is currently widely used.[19] Patients with high-grade transformation of EMC are older than typical EMC cases, with an average age of 76 years of age.[22] This tumor demonstrates a more aggressive biological behavior than others, showing more frequent extraglandular extension, lymph node metastasis, and distant metastasis than typical EMC.[22]

Immunohistochemically, luminal ductal cells are strongly positive for epithelial markers, including pan-cytokeratin (CK) (AE1/AE3), low-molecular-weight CK (CAM5.2), and CK7 (**Fig.** 1C), whereas abluminal myoepithelial cells are negative to weakly positive for these markers.[1,4] Among various myoepithelial markers, α-smooth muscle actin (**Fig.** 1D) is highly sensitive and specific for myoepithelial cells, whereas S100 protein and p63/p40 are less specific, and calponin is less sensitive.[1] The Ki-67 labeling index varies widely among cases, from 0% to 70%, with a mean of 16.9% to 20.5%.[1,4]

CYTOLOGY

Fine needle aspiration of EMC is usually cellular and characterized by the presence of epithelial cells and clear myoepithelial cells (**Fig.** 3A, B). Epithelial cells are smaller, darker cells showing cohesive sheets or sometimes tubular structures. Myoepithelial cells are larger cells with clear or scant cytoplasm, and they are less cohesive than epithelial cells and often dispersed (see **Fig.** 3B).[23–25] These 2 cellular components are not readily distinguishable in some cases.[23] Because the myoepithelial cells are fragile, the cytoplasm is easily disrupted by mechanical forces during smearing, so naked nuclei of myoepithelial cells can be predominant in fine needle aspiration findings (see **Fig.** 3A).[23–25] Hyaline stromal material is sometimes observed.[24] When the globular form of hyaline material is present, the aspirate closely resembles AdCC.[9]

MOLECULAR PATHOLOGY FEATURES

HRAS hotspot point mutations analyzed by Sanger and/or next-generation sequencing have

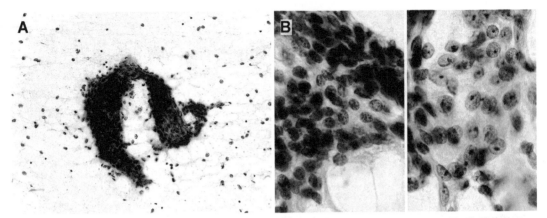

Fig. 3. Fine needle aspirate of EMC. Cohesive luminal ductal cells form tubular structures with disrupted myoepithelial cells often presenting as naked nuclei in the background (*A*). Luminal ductal cells have uniformly round nuclei with a relatively high nuclear cytoplasmic ratio (*B, left*). Myoepithelial cells have larger nuclei than luminal ductal cells and abundant pale cytoplasm (*B, right*).

been reported in EMC.[16,17,26–28] The mutation frequency reportedly ranges from 26.7% to 81.7%.[4,16,17] The most common mutation site is codon 61 (Q61R), but other mutation patterns (G13R, Q61K) are also identified.[4,16,17] No significant correlation has been found between the *HRAS* mutation status and histologic variations or other histologic aggressiveness, such as nuclear grade, the presence of necrosis, lymphovascular invasion, perineural invasion, the mitotic count, or the Ki-67 labeling index.[4] Of note, the *HRAS* mutation was not detected in any other salivary gland tumor entities manifesting EMC-like features, including AdCC, PA, BCA/BCAC, and myoepithelial carcinoma with clear myoepithelial cells.[4] Therefore, the assessment of *HRAS* mutations is a useful molecular test for diagnosing EMC to discriminate it from its histologic mimics.[4] Identical *HRAS* mutations have also been identified in 13% to 27% of salivary duct carcinoma cases.[27,29–32] However, salivary duct carcinoma shows marked nuclear atypia without biphasic differentiation and is not usually included in the differential diagnosis of EMC. In addition, a minority of EMC cases harbor *PIK3CA* and *AKT1* mutations, regardless of the presence of *HRAS* mutations.[4,17,27] A recent case report revealed heterogeneous *ARID1A* loss and terminating mutations in an EMC with an extensive solid oncocytic differentiation.[33]

DIAGNOSIS

The diagnosis of EMC exhibiting entirely classical histologic features is relatively straightforward; however, the histologic variety and the clear cell morphology discussed elsewhere in this article in

other tumor entities can complicate the accurate diagnosis of EMC.

There are 3 steps for diagnosing of EMC. First, confirm the malignant nature of the tumor. The invasive tumor border, considerable nuclear atypia, coagulative necrosis, conspicuous mitotic activity, and perineural and lymphovascular invasion may be findings suggestive of malignancy. However, an ill-defined highly infiltrative growth is unusual in EMC, and many are well-circumscribed with minimal invasion, and PA conversely sometimes show capsular and extracapsular extension.[1,34] Therefore, the evaluation of the tumor border is not necessarily easy. A multilobular manner of invasion is relatively characteristic of EMC.[1] Mitotic figures are usually found in fewer than 5 of 10 high-power fields, and the majority of cases lack necrosis and lymphovascular invasion.[1,4]

Second, check for any biphasic differentiation in the tumor. Myoepithelial cells overgrow luminal ductal cells in most cases. Furthermore, in double clear EMC, luminal ductal cells are difficult to recognize. In such cases, immunohistochemical staining using epithelial and myoepithelial markers helps to identify hidden epithelial components. A normal salivary duct trapped within the tumor should not be misinterpreted as a neoplastic duct.

Third, look for clear myoepithelial cells. The presence of luminal ductal cells surrounded by clear myoepithelial cells is the definition of EMC. The clear cytoplasm of myoepithelial cells may be difficult to recognize owing to the large nuclear/cytoplasmic ratio.

The final diagnosis of EMC should ideally be made by using resected samples with tumor borders. Information on the invasive front, predominant growth pattern, the presence of biphasic differentiation, and cytomorphology can facilitate the diagnosis. The diagnosis can be made by a core needle biopsy; however, the cautious exclusion of other tumor types is necessary because of the indeterminate nature of the tumor boundary. It is usually difficult and not recommended to diagnose EMC using fine needle aspiration alone. Because the differential diagnoses include many benign to malignant tumors, fine needle aspiration would be classified in salivary gland neoplasm of uncertain malignant potential or suspicious for malignancy categories in the Milan System for Reporting Salivary Gland Cytopathology.[35] Intraoperative frozen sections are even more difficult to use for a diagnosis. Myoepithelial cells, in general, can be easily affected by a tissue-processing artifact and misleadingly tend to become having clear cytoplasm seen in EMC.

The main role of immunohistochemical staining in the diagnosis of EMC is to verify the biphasic nature of the tumor and assess the cell proliferative activity. Sanger sequencing to detect HRAS mutations is useful for confirming the diagnosis, given its high sensitivity and specificity.[4]

DIFFERENTIAL DIAGNOSIS

The differential diagnoses of EMC include salivary gland tumors showing myoepithelial differentiation with or without ductal formation and those consisting of clear cells, such as AdCC, BCA/BCAC, PA, myoepithelial carcinoma, clear cell carcinoma, sebaceous adenocarcinoma, clear cell variant of mucoepidermoid and acinic cell carcinomas, and metastatic renal cell carcinoma (Table 1). Particularly challenging cases may require not only the careful evaluation of certain histomorphologic characteristics of each tumor, but also the use of ancillary tests of immunohistochemistry and molecular analyses.

ADENOID CYSTIC CARCINOMA

The differential diagnosis between EMC and AdCC is the most problematic issue, because they often share architectural and cytologic features, at least focally, and even are sometimes absolutely indistinguishable.[8,9] Both are carcinomas with biphasic ductal and myoepithelial differentiation and can exhibit similar cribriform, tubular, and trabecular patterns. Because the multinodular and encapsulated types of invasive front are common in EMC, accounting for 87% of cases, tumors with highly infiltrative borders accompanied by perineural

invasion tend to be AdCC instead of EMC. Although, like EMC, the myoepithelial cells of AdCC occasionally have clear cytoplasm (Fig. 4A), they are basaloid in appearance and possess hyperchromatic angulated nuclei with indistinct nucleoli, whereas those of EMC have plump oval nuclei with open chromatin.

The KIT and MYB immunohistochemical expression may be characteristic of AdCC, but can also be found in EMC, and the specificity is not necessarily high.[8,36] However, because most AdCCs specifically show MYB or MYBL1 rearrangement, a fluorescence in situ hybridization analysis is useful for diagnosing AdCC, whereas the detection of HRAS hotspot mutations by Sanger sequencing can help to confirm the diagnosis of EMC.[4]

BASAL CELL ADENOMA AND ADENOCARCINOMA

BCA/BCAC are also biphasic salivary gland tumors, and their composition of clear myoepithelial cells may resemble EMC with basaloid features (Fig. 4B). A jigsaw puzzle–like histologic pattern together with β-catenin nuclear immunoexpression and the presence of S100 protein-positive stromal spindle cells is suggestive of BCA/BCAC.[37,38] In addition, BCA/BCAC and EMC specifically harbor CTNNB1 and HRAS point mutations, respectively.[39,40]

PLEOMORPHIC ADENOMA

When the characteristic myxochondroid matrix is evident, the diagnosis of PA is relatively easy; however, cellular PA can be difficult to distinguish from EMC. Similar to EMC, myoepithelial cells in PA sometimes have clear cytoplasm, and some authors insist that the line between cellular PA and encapsulated EMC can be difficult to draw (Fig. 4C).[1] Although PA is a well-circumscribed benign tumor, a considerable percentage (26% and 40%) of PA cases shows capsule penetration and even extension through the capsule, which can be misinterpreted as invasion of EMC.[34]

The major difference between these 2 tumors is the nuclear size and atypia. The tumor cell nuclei of EMC are larger than those of PA and have atypia compatible with malignancy, albeit mild to moderate in general. The specificity of PLAG1 and HMGA2 immunohistochemistry for discriminating PA from EMC is controversial.[41–43] However, a fluorescence in situ hybridization analysis for PLAG1 and HMGA2 rearrangements can be a useful diagnostic tool for PA.

Table 1
Differential diagnosis

	Epithelial-Myoepithelial Carcinoma	Adenoid Cystic Carcinoma	Basal Cell Adenoma	Basal Cell Adenocarcinoma	Pleomorphic adenoma	Myoepithelial Carcinoma	Clear Cell Carcinoma
Biological behavior	Low-grade malignancy	Intermediate grade malignancy	Benign	Low-grade malignancy	Benign	Intermediate grade malignancy	Low-grade malignancy
Location	Parotid gland (majority)	Major salivary glands > minor salivary glands	Parotid gland (majority)	Parotid gland (majority)	Major salivary glands > minor salivary glands	Major salivary glands > minor salivary glands	Minor salivary glands (mostly)
Tumor border	Minimally invasive	Highly infiltrative	Well-circumscribed and encapsulated	Lobular pattern of invasion	Well-circumscribed and encapsulated; occasional capsular or extracapsular extension	Infiltrative	Unencapsulated, infiltrative
Growth pattern	Multilobular, bilayered tubular, trabecular, solid, cribriform	Cribriform, tubular, solid	Solid with peripheral palisading, tubular, trabecular	Solid with peripheral palisading, tubular, trabecular	Bilayered tubular, myxochondroid stroma	Solid, reticular, myxoid, hyalinized stroma	Solid, nest, trabecular, sheet; hyalinized stroma
Cytomorphology	Eosinophilic ductal cells + clear myoepithelial cells (mild to moderate atypia)	Hyperchromatic angulated nuclei (mild to moderate atypia)	Basaloid (bland)	Basaloid (mild atypia)	Variable (bland)	Epithelioid, spindle, plasmacytoid, clear (moderate atypia)	Clear (mild atypia)
Biphasic ductal and myoepithelial differentiation	(+)	(+)	(+)	(+)	(+)	(−)	(−)

Characteristic immunohistochemical staining	Specific myoepithelial marker (+)	Specific myoepithelial marker (+), MYB (+)	Specific myoepithelial marker (+), β-catenin (nuclear +), S100 (+) stromal spindle cells	Specific myoepithelial marker (+), β-catenin (nuclear +), S100 (+) stromal spindle cells	Specific myoepithelial marker (+), PLAG1 (+), HMGA2 (+)	Specific myoepithelial marker (+) / Specific myoepithelial marker (−)
Molecular genetics	HRAS mutations (85%)	MYB/MYBL1-NFIB fusion (~100%)	CTNNB1 mutation (60%)	CTNNB1 mutation (40%)	PLAG1/HMGA2 rearrangement (75%)	EWSR1 rearrangement (clear cell variant) / EWSR1-ATF1 fusion (90%)

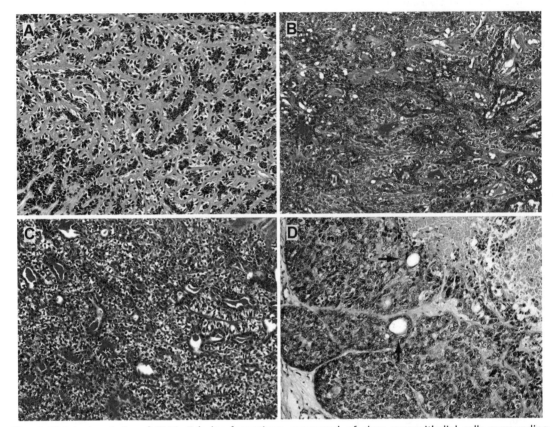

Fig. 4. Histologic mimics of EMC. Tubular formations, composed of clear myoepithelial cells surrounding epithelial-lined ductal cells, in adenoid cystic carcinoma (*A*), basal cell adenoma (*B*), and pleomorphic adenoma (*C*). (*D*) Myoepithelial carcinoma-like carcinoma with limited foci of ductal differentiation. The tumor is predominantly composed of myoepithelial cells with high-grade atypical nuclei as well as scant cytoplasm without obvious clarity, which differs from the finding of typical EMC. A few ductal epithelial cells are also observed (*arrows*).

MYOEPITHELIAL CARCINOMA AND CLEAR CELL CARCINOMA

Distinguishing between myoepithelial carcinoma and EMC is principally based on the presence or absence of true ductal formation. Myoepithelial carcinoma composed predominantly of a clear cell component can be difficult to distinguish from EMC with myoepithelial cell overgrowth (see **Fig. 1E**). Epithelial markers are useful for highlighting luminal ductal cells in EMC, which show a stronger expression than myoepithelial cells (**Fig. 1F**). Furthermore, involvement of normal salivary ducts must be carefully eliminated.

Tumors almost entirely composed of myoepithelial cells with high-grade nuclear atypia and a few ductal cells were categorized as myoepithelial carcinoma in the third edition of Armed Forces Institute of Pathology Fascicle, but they were removed from that category in the latest version.[44,45] A recent report designated such tumors as "myoepithelial carcinoma-like carcinoma with limited foci of ductal differentiation" (**Fig. 4D**) because of the lack of clear myoepithelial cells and an *HRAS* mutation.[4]

Clear cell carcinoma is devoid of the myoepithelial differentiation of EMC and shows a negative immunoreaction for α-smooth muscle actin and calponin, although positivity may be found for p40 and p63. In contrast with the preponderance of the major salivary glands as the site of EMC, clear cell carcinomas almost exclusively arise in the intraoral minor salivary glands.[46] Genetically, most clear cell carcinomas characteristically carry the *EWSR1-ATF1* fusion gene.[47,48]

PROGNOSIS

EMC basically behaves indolently, with 5- and 10-year disease-specific survivals of 93.5% and

81.8%, respectively.[1] Although local recurrence does occasionally occur (in 30%–50% of patients), lymph node and distant metastases are rare.[1,49,50] Significant prognostic factors have been reported to include the margin status, lymphovascular invasion, tumor necrosis, and high-grade transformation, including myoepithelial anaplasia.[1,3]

The histologic variations may not affect the patient survival. Although only a limited number of cases collected include survival data, EMC with high-grade transformation generally follows a more aggressive course with a poorer prognosis than typical EMC.[1,6,18]

SUMMARY

EMC is one of the most challenging salivary gland tumor types to diagnose. Recent reports have shed light on its histologic variations and molecular genetics. Careful inspection of the whole specimen is essential in the differential diagnosis, and ancillary immunohistochemical and molecular tests can contribute to the correct diagnosis.

CLINICS CARE POINTS

- EMC is a low-grade salivary gland carcinoma characterized by biphasic tubular structures composed of inner ductal and outer clear myoepithelial cells.
- Distinction from other benign and malignant tumor is essential but often challenging.
- High-grade transformation is rare but associated with a poor prognosis.

DISCLOSURE

The authors have nothing to disclose.

REFERENCES

1. Seethala RR, Barnes EL, Hunt JL. Epithelial-myoepithelial carcinoma: a review of the clinicopathologic spectrum and immunophenotypic characteristics in 61 tumors of the salivary glands and upper aerodigestive tract. Am J Surg Pathol 2007;31(1):44–57.
2. Epithelial-myoepithelial carcinoma. In: Ellis G, Auclair P, editors. Tumors of the salivary glands (AFIP atlas of tumor pathology: series 4). Washington, DC: American Registry of Pathology; 2008. p. 309–22.
3. Seethala R, Bell D, Fonseca I, et al. Epithelial-myoepithelial carcinoma. In: El-Naggar AK, Chan JKC, Grandis JR, et al, editors. WHO classification of head and neck tumours. Lyon (France): International Agency for Research on Cancer; 2017.
4. Urano M, Nakaguro M, Yamamoto Y, et al. Diagnostic significance of HRAS mutations in epithelial-myoepithelial carcinomas exhibiting a broad histopathologic spectrum. Am J Surg Pathol 2019; 43(7):984–94.
5. Donath K, Seifert G, Schmitz R. Diagnosis and ultrastructure of the tubular carcinoma of salivary gland ducts. Epithelial-myoepithelial carcinoma of the intercalated ducts. Virchows Arch A Pathol Pathol Anat 1972;356(1):16–31.
6. Fonseca I, Soares J. Epithelial-myoepithelial carcinoma of the salivary glands. A study of 22 cases. Virchows Arch A Pathol Anat Histopathol 1993; 422(5):389–96.
7. Daley TD, Wysocki GP, Smout MS, et al. Epithelial-myoepithelial carcinoma of salivary glands. Oral Surg Oral Med Oral Pathol 1984;57(5):512–9.
8. Bishop JA, Westra WH. MYB translocation status in salivary gland epithelial-myoepithelial carcinoma: evaluation of classic, variant, and hybrid forms. Am J Surg Pathol 2018;42(3):319–25.
9. Aisagbonhi OA, Tulecke MA, Wilbur DC, et al. Fine-needle aspiration of epithelial-myoepithelial carcinoma of the parotid gland with prominent adenoid cystic carcinoma-like cribriform features: avoiding a diagnostic pitfall. Am J Clin Pathol 2016;146(6): 741–6.
10. Seethala RR. Basaloid/blue salivary gland tumors. Mod Pathol 2017;30(s1):S84–95.
11. Shinozaki A, Nagao T, Endo H, et al. Sebaceous epithelial-myoepithelial carcinoma of the salivary gland: clinicopathologic and immunohistochemical analysis of 6 cases of a new histologic variant. Am J Surg Pathol 2008;32(6):913–23.
12. Seethala RR. Oncocytic and apocrine epithelial myoepithelial carcinoma: novel variants of a challenging tumor. Head Neck Pathol 2013;7:S77–84. Suppl 1(Suppl 1).
13. Seethala RR, Richmond JA, Hoschar AP, et al. New variants of epithelial-myoepithelial carcinoma: oncocytic-sebaceous and apocrine. Arch Pathol Lab Med 2009;133(6):950–9.
14. Hussaini HM, Angel CM, Speight PM, et al. A double-clear variant of epithelial-myoepithelial carcinoma of the parotid gland. Head Neck Pathol 2012;6(4):471–5.
15. Hellquist H, Skalova A, Azadeh B. Salivary gland hybrid tumour revisited: could they represent high-grade transformation in a low-grade neoplasm? Virchows Arch 2016;469(6):643–50.
16. Chiosea SI, Miller M, Seethala RR. HRAS mutations in epithelial-myoepithelial carcinoma. Head Neck Pathol 2014;8(2):146–50.
17. El Hallani S, Udager AM, Bell D, et al. Epithelial-myoepithelial carcinoma: frequent morphologic

and molecular evidence of preexisting pleomorphic adenoma, common HRAS mutations in PLAG1-intact and HMGA2-intact cases, and occasional TP53, FBXW7, and SMARCB1 alterations in high-grade cases. Am J Surg Pathol 2018;42(1):18–27.

18. Alos L, Carrillo R, Ramos J, et al. High-grade carcinoma component in epithelial-myoepithelial carcinoma of salivary glands clinicopathological, immunohistochemical and flow-cytometric study of three cases. Virchows Arch 1999;434(4):291–9.

19. Roy P, Bullock MJ, Perez-Ordoñez B, et al. Epithelial-myoepithelial carcinoma with high grade transformation. Am J Surg Pathol 2010;34(9):1258–65.

20. Fonseca I, Félix A, Soares J. Dedifferentiation in salivary gland carcinomas. Am J Surg Pathol 2000;24(3):469–71.

21. Kusafuka K, Takizawa Y, Ueno T, et al. Dedifferentiated epithelial-myoepithelial carcinoma of the parotid gland: a rare case report of immunohistochemical analysis and review of the literature. Oral Surg Oral Med Oral Pathol Oral Radiol Endod 2008;106(1):85–91.

22. Nagao T. "Dedifferentiation" and high-grade transformation in salivary gland carcinomas. Head Neck Pathol 2013;7:S37–47. Suppl 1(Suppl 1).

23. Miliauskas JR, Orell SR. Fine-needle aspiration cytological findings in five cases of epithelial-myoepithelial carcinoma of salivary glands. Diagn Cytopathol 2003;28(3):163–7.

24. Molnar SL, Zarka MA, De Las Casas LE. Going beyond "basaloid neoplasm": fine needle aspiration cytology of epithelial-myoepithelial carcinoma of the parotid gland. Diagn Cytopathol 2016;44(5):422–5.

25. Arora VK, Misra K, Bhatia A. Cytomorphologic features of the rare epithelial-myoepithelial carcinoma of the salivary gland. Acta Cytol 1990;34(2):239–42.

26. Cros J, Sbidian E, Hans S, et al. Expression and mutational status of treatment-relevant targets and key oncogenes in 123 malignant salivary gland tumours. Ann Oncol 2013;24(10):2624–9.

27. Grunewald I, Vollbrecht C, Meinrath J, et al. Targeted next generation sequencing of parotid gland cancer uncovers genetic heterogeneity. Oncotarget 2015;6(20):18224–37.

28. Prior IA, Lewis PD, Mattos C. A comprehensive survey of ras mutations in cancer. Cancer Res 2012;72(10):2457–67.

29. Luk PP, Weston JD, Yu B, et al. Salivary duct carcinoma: clinicopathologic features, morphologic spectrum, and somatic mutations. Head Neck 2016;38(Suppl 1):E1838–47.

30. Dalin MG, Desrichard A, Katabi N, et al. Comprehensive molecular characterization of salivary duct carcinoma reveals actionable targets and similarity to apocrine breast cancer. Clin Cancer Res 2016;22(18):4623–33.

31. Chiosea SI, Williams L, Griffith CC, et al. Molecular characterization of apocrine salivary duct carcinoma. Am J Surg Pathol 2015;39(6):744–52.

32. Shimura T, Tada Y, Hirai H, et al. Prognostic and histogenetic roles of gene alteration and the expression of key potentially actionable targets in salivary duct carcinomas. Oncotarget 2018;9(2):1852–67.

33. Rupp NJ, Brada M, Skálová A, et al. New insights into tumor heterogeneity: a case of solid-oncocytic epithelial-myoepithelial carcinoma of the parotid gland harboring a HRAS and heterogeneous terminating ARID1A mutation. Head Neck Pathol 2020;4(2):554–8.

34. Zbären P, Stauffer E. Pleomorphic adenoma of the parotid gland: histopathologic analysis of the capsular characteristics of 218 tumors. Head Neck 2007;29(8):751–7.

35. Faquin WC, Rossi ED, Baloch Z, et al. The Milan system for reporting salivary gland cytopathology. Cham, Switzerland: Springer; 2018.

36. Andreadis D, Epivatianos A, Poulopoulos A, et al. Detection of C-KIT (CD117) molecule in benign and malignant salivary gland tumours. Oral Oncol 2006;42(1):57–65.

37. Kawahara A, Harada H, Abe H, et al. Nuclear β-catenin expression in basal cell adenomas of salivary gland. J Oral Pathol Med 2011;40(6):460–6.

38. Dardick I, Daley TD, van Nostrand AW. Basal cell adenoma with myoepithelial cell-derived "stroma": a new major salivary gland tumor entity. Head Neck Surg 1986;8(4):257–67.

39. Sato M, Yamamoto H, Hatanaka Y, et al. Wnt/β-catenin signal alteration and its diagnostic utility in basal cell adenoma and histologically similar tumors of the salivary gland. Pathol Res Pract 2018;214(4):586–92.

40. Jo VY, Sholl LM, Krane JF. Distinctive patterns of CTNNB1 (β-Catenin) alterations in salivary gland basal cell adenoma and basal cell adenocarcinoma. Am J Surg Pathol 2016;40(8):1143–50.

41. de Brito BS, Giovanelli N, Egal ES, et al. Loss of expression of Plag1 in malignant transformation from pleomorphic adenoma to carcinoma ex pleomorphic adenoma. Hum Pathol 2016;57:152–9.

42. Rotellini M, Palomba A, Baroni G, et al. Diagnostic utility of PLAG1 immunohistochemical determination in salivary gland tumors. Appl Immunohistochem Mol Morphol 2014;22(5):390–4.

43. Mito JK, Jo VY, Chiosea SI, et al. HMGA2 is a specific immunohistochemical marker for pleomorphic adenoma and carcinoma ex-pleomorphic adenoma. Histopathology 2017;71(4):511–21.

44. Ellis GL, Auclair P. Tumors of the salivary glands (AFIP atlas of tumor pathology; 3rd series).

Washington, DC: Armed Forces Institute of Pathology; 1996.

45. Ellis GL, Auclair P. Tumors of the salivary glands (AFIP atlas of tumor pathology: series 4). Washington, DC: American Registry of Pathology; 2008.

46. Daniele L, Nikolarakos D, Keenan J, et al. Clear cell carcinoma, not otherwise specified/hyalinising clear cell carcinoma of the salivary gland: the current nomenclature, clinical/pathological characteristics and management. Crit Rev Oncol Hematol 2016; 102:55–64.

47. Skálová A, Weinreb I, Hyrcza M, et al. Clear cell myoepithelial carcinoma of salivary glands showing EWSR1 rearrangement: molecular analysis of 94 salivary gland carcinomas with prominent clear cell component. Am J Surg Pathol 2015;39(3):338–48.

48. Antonescu CR, Katabi N, Zhang L, et al. EWSR1-ATF1 fusion is a novel and consistent finding in hyalinizing clear-cell carcinoma of salivary gland. Genes Chromosomes Cancer 2011;50(7):559–70.

49. Gore MR. Epithelial-myoepithelial carcinoma: a population-based survival analysis. BMC Ear Nose Throat Disord 2018;18:15.

50. Vázquez A, Patel TD, D'Aguillo CM, et al. Epithelial-myoepithelial carcinoma of the salivary glands: an analysis of 246 cases. Otolaryngol Head Neck Surg 2015;153(4):569–74.

Salivary Duct Carcinoma
An Aggressive Salivary Gland Carcinoma with Morphologic Variants, Newly Identified Molecular Characteristics, and Emerging Treatment Modalities

Mobeen Rahman, MD[a,b],
Christopher C. Griffith, MD, PhD[a,b],*

KEYWORDS

• Salivary duct carcinoma • Apocrine • Androgen receptor • Salivary gland • Molecular

Key points

- Salivary duct carcinoma is one of the most aggressive salivary gland malignancies and is associated with significant mortality.

- Salivary duct carcinoma is characterized by apocrine morphology, even focally in cases where there is variant morphology.

- Most salivary duct carcinomas show a unique immunophenotype: androgen receptor positive/gross cystic disease fluid protein positive/estrogen receptor negative/progesterone receptor negative.

- Although no standardized treatment regimen exists for salivary duct carcinoma, treatment commonly includes complete surgical excision with lymph node dissection and postoperative radiation with or without chemotherapy.

- Continued study is examining the efficacy of regimens involving androgen deprivation therapy and/or molecular targets in salivary duct carcinoma.

ABSTRACT

Salivary duct carcinoma (SDC) is a rare, aggressive salivary gland malignancy with significant mortality. Morphologically, most tumors are characterized by apocrine differentiation with a typical immunophenotype of androgen receptor positive/gross cystic disease fluid protein positive/estrogen receptor negative/progesterone receptor negative. Several morphologic variants of SDC exist, representing diagnostic pitfalls. Several differential diagnoses should be considered because prognosis, treatment, and management may be different from SDC. For SDC, current treatment strategies are aggressive and commonly include surgical excision with lymph node dissection and adjuvant radiotherapy. Continued research is examining the utility of androgen deprivation therapy and targeted molecular therapy.

OVERVIEW

The original description of salivary duct carcinoma (SDC) is attributed to Kleinsasser and colleagues[1]

[a] The Robert J. Tomsich Pathology and Laboratory Medicine Institute, Cleveland Clinic, Cleveland, OH, USA;
[b] Cleveland Clinic Head and Neck Pathology, Mail Code L25, 9500 Euclid Avenue, Cleveland, OH 44195, USA
* Corresponding author. Cleveland Clinic Head and Neck Pathology, Mail Code L25, 9500 Euclid Avenue, Cleveland, OH 44195.
E-mail address: griffic8@ccf.org
Twitter: @ENT_path (M.R.)

Surgical Pathology 14 (2021) 111–126
https://doi.org/10.1016/j.path.2020.09.010

in 1968, in which they described a novel group of parotid gland malignancies morphologically similar to mammary ductal carcinoma. In 1991, SDC was included in the second edition of the World Health Organization (WHO) classification of salivary gland tumors for the first time.[2,3] Since that time, understanding of this entity has grown. Two important studies by Dr Leon Barnes and colleagues in 2000 and 2001 noted that SDC had a close immunophenotypic similarity to prostatic carcinoma, had specific morphologic characteristics, and frequently expressed androgen receptor (AR).[4–6] Continued molecular characterization of this aggressive malignancy has taken place with the goal to identify and develop new therapeutic and prognostic markers.

In general, SDC is an aggressive malignancy commonly associated with metastases, local recurrence, and significant mortality. These tumors have a predilection for men (male/female, 5.5:1)[7,8] and most frequently involve the parotid gland, followed by the submandibular gland.[7,9] There is a broad age range at presentation (22–91 years), but the tumor preferentially occurs in older patients (mean, 60–79 years) and is uncommon in patients less than 50 years old.[9] SDC is uncommon, representing only approximately 10% of all salivary gland malignancies.[8] The clinical course can be rapid and advanced at initial presentation, with most patients presenting with lymph node metastases (up to 83%).[2,7] Local recurrence occurs in up to 40% of patients and distant metastases are common (up to 66%).[7] Accurate diagnosis is important for proper counseling and management of patients, identification of potential markers for therapeutic interventions, and continued investigation into new treatment modalities.

GROSS FEATURES

The gross findings of SDC frequently reflect the aggressive nature of this tumor but are otherwise nonspecific. SDC commonly shows an ill-defined border with infiltration of adjacent parenchyma (Fig. 1). A gritty cut surface is common. There may be areas of cystic change, necrosis, or hemorrhage.[5] Tumor size varies, ranging from 1.0 cm to more than 5.5 cm with a mean of 2.9 cm.[4] If a nodal dissection is also performed, lymph node metastases are common and may be recognized grossly. A residual pleomorphic adenoma (PA) may be grossly identified in some patients with variable proportions of SDC and PA. When the possibility of carcinoma arising in a PA (ie, carcinoma ex-PA) is suspected, extensive sampling may be required to confirm malignancy and determine the extent of invasion depending on the proportion of carcinoma (more issues related to SDC ex-PA are discussed later).

MICROSCOPIC FEATURES

SDC is a high-grade adenocarcinoma of the salivary glands with apocrine differentiation.[6,10] High-grade cytologic features are usually obvious, with pleomorphic nuclei having coarse chromatin and prominent nucleoli (Fig. 2A).[9,11] Nuclear pleomorphism is frequently marked, but in some cases more uniform nuclear enlargement can hinder the recognition of this significant nuclear enlargement.[2,9] Large, so-called cherry-red nucleoli are also commonly present. Prominent mitotic activity and atypical mitotic figures can usually be found. Necrosis, particularly comedo-type necrosis, is present in many patients (Fig. 2B). A variety of growth patterns can be seen, including solid, cystic, and papillary.[9] Morphologic evidence of apocrine differentiation, including apocrine snouts and secretions, can be seen in many patients but may be only focal (Fig. 2C). Abundant eosinophilic, granular, vacuolated, or foamy cytoplasm is present in almost all patients as a result of apocrine differentiation. An in situ component (representing encapsulated carcinoma ex-PA or intraductal carcinoma) may be identified in some patients (Fig. 2D). Even when invasive, SDCs commonly have areas with well-defined nests with cribriform architecture, Roman bridge–like structures, and comedo-type necrosis imparting the appearance of ductal carcinoma in situ (DCIS) of breast.[7] In some patients, a truly in situ component can be subtle when the invasive component is extensive.[10] SDC is commonly associated with lymphovascular and perineural invasion.[9] Several morphologic variants of SDC have been described, and these are discussed next.

MICROPAPILLARY VARIANT

As in adenocarcinomas arising in other organ systems, micropapillary architecture can be seen in SDC.[12] This variant is uncommon, with varying incidence from 3.7% to 17%.[11,13] Micropapillary architecture is characterized by small clusters of cells without central fibrovascular cores in clear spaces (Fig. 3A).[12,13] The cells have moderate-grade to high-grade nuclear features with large and conspicuous nucleoli and readily identifiable mitoses. Psammoma bodies are typically not identified and mucin stains are typically negative.[12] Compared with typical SDC and other variants, micropapillary SDC is associated with a worse prognosis, possibly related to higher rates of

Fig. 1. Gross view of SDC arising from the parotid gland. Note the invasive nature of the tumor with gross extraparotid spread to involve subcutaneous tissue. (*Courtesy of* K. Magliocca, DDS, MPH, Atlanta, GA.)

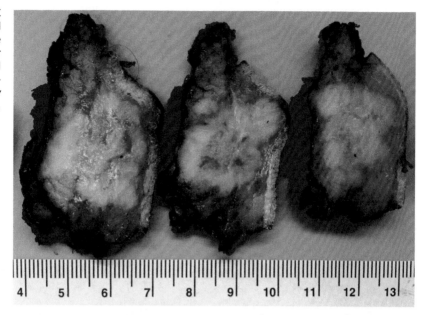

perineural invasion, lymphovascular invasion, and lymph node metastases.[10,13] In their series of micropapillary SDC, Luk and colleagues[13] reported a median survival of only 9 months, compared with 56 months for a conventional SDC. Micropapillary architecture can be found in varying proportion and it is unclear how much is required for designation as a variant. However, given the worse prognosis, the presence of an invasive micropapillary component in SDC should be noted when identified.[10,12,13]

MUCINOUS VARIANT

The original description of a mucinous variant was presented in a series by Simpson and colleagues[14] in 2003. In most cases, a conventional SDC component is identified, although a pure mucinous SDC has been described.[14,15] In all cases, there are small clusters or single cells, occasionally including signet ring cells, floating in pools of abundant mucin.[14] Similar to conventional SDC, tumor cells maintain high-grade nuclear features and abundant eosinophilic cytoplasm even in areas of extensive mucinous differentiation. The differential diagnosis for mucinous SDC includes high-grade mucoepidermoid carcinoma (MEC) and metastases. MECs are typically positive for p63, whereas SDCs are negative.[2] In contrast, AR is positive in almost all SDCs and is only positive in a small subset of MECs (up to 5%).[16] Although mucinous variants of carcinoma in other organ sites tend to have better prognosis (ie,

breast) the mucinous variant of SDC is associated with aggressive clinical behavior similar to its conventional counterpart.[14]

SARCOMATOID VARIANT

Sarcomatoid SDC is diagnosed when there is a dimorphic pattern of both conventional SDC and a sarcomatous component, with or without heterologous components.[10,17] A transition zone between the 2 components can be found in some instances.[17] In sarcomatoid areas, highly atypical spindle cells are commonly arranged in a fascicular pattern (**Fig.** 3B, C). Tumor cells are enlarged and hyperchromatic, and atypical mitotic forms are common.[6] Bizarre malignant, multinucleated cells and occasional rhabdoid cells may be present.[17] Immunohistochemistry (IHC) can confirm the epithelial nature of the sarcomatoid component in some patients.[9] Heterologous deposition of malignant osteoid material has also been described but is of no known significance.[10,17] The differential diagnosis includes carcinosarcoma and a true sarcoma if a conventional SDC component is not sampled or recognized.[10] Sarcomatoid SDC is an aggressive malignancy; however, overall survival is not significantly different than conventional SDC.[17]

ONCOCYTIC VARIANT

SDC is generally oncocytoid as a result of abundant eosinophilic cytoplasm, but a truly oncocytic

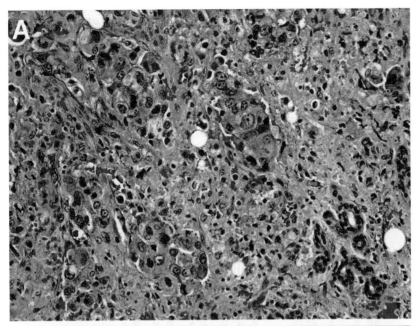

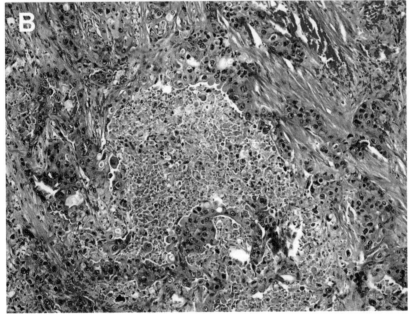

Fig. 2. Histomorphology of SDC. (*A*) SDC is a prototypical high-grade adenocarcinoma showing tumor cells with enlarged pleomorphic nuclei, prominent nucleoli, and abundant eosinophilic cytoplasm. Note the benign ductal structures in lower right for comparison (hematoxylin-eosin [H&E], original magnification ×200). (*B*) Comedo-type necrosis is a common finding (H&E, original magnification ×100).

variant of SDC also occurs. To classify a tumor as oncocytic variant SDC, an arbitrary cutoff of greater than 50% truly oncocytic tumor cells has been defined in the literature.[10] This variant has enlarged but less pleomorphic nuclei with less robust desmoplasia. Tumor cells have abundant, finely granular cytoplasm containing centrally placed nuclei and single prominent nucleoli (**Fig. 3**D). Classic areas of conventional SDC can be sparse and ample sampling of the tumor may be required.[2] Perineural and lymphovascular invasion can be found as well as tumor-associated lymphoid proliferations.[2] The differential diagnosis includes oncocytic MEC, oncocytic carcinoma, acinic cell carcinoma (AciCC), and metastatic breast carcinoma. An IHC panel consisting of AR, GATA3, p63, and DOG1 can be helpful because most SDCs are positive for AR and GATA3 but negative for p63 and DOG1.[2] Clinical

Fig. 2. (continued). (C) Apocrine differentiation is an important defining feature of SDC. Morphologic evidence of apocrine differentiation includes apocrine snouts as seen in the luminal aspects of this focus (H&E, original magnification ×100). (D) Areas of invasive SDC can have an appearance reminiscent of high-grade ductal carcinoma of the breast with central comedotype necrosis and cribriform/Roman-bridge architecture (H&E, original magnification ×100).

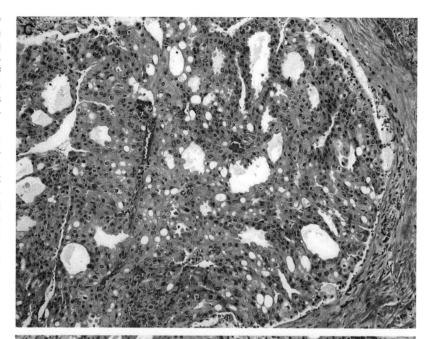

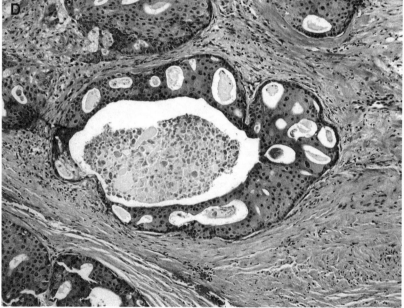

correlation is also helpful if metastasis from a breast primary is considered.

BASAL-LIKE VARIANT

The basal-like variant of SDC is diagnostically challenging and descriptions of this variant are limited in the literature. Areas of conventional SDC may be limited to areas of a preexisting PA with the invasive component showing basaloid morphology.[6] These basaloid areas have less abundant and more amphophilic cytoplasm compared with conventional SDC. p63, CK5/6, and epidermal growth factor receptor (EGFR) expression can be detected in basaloid areas with loss of AR expression.[11,18] Because of these morphologic and immunophenotypic differences, extensive sampling may be needed to recognize the basal-like variant of SDC, particularly because most cases in the literature have minimal conventional SDC components.[6,11]

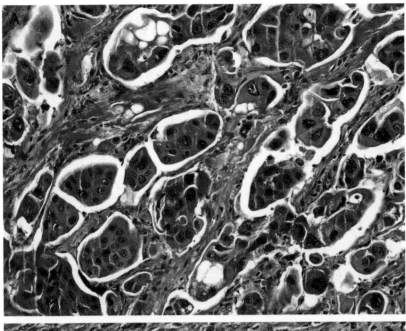

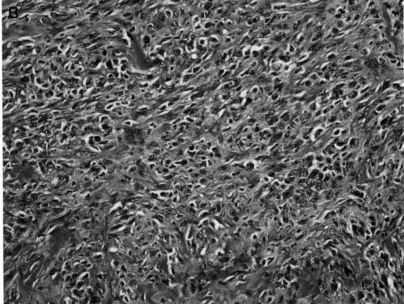

Fig. 3. Variant morphologies of SDC are important to recognize. (*A*) Micropapillary SDC shows small clusters of high-grade tumor cells lacking fibrovascular cores and having prominent separation from surrounding stroma (H&E, original magnification ×200). (*B,*

SALIVARY DUCT CARCINOMA EX PLEOMORPHIC ADENOMA

As noted previously, SDC commonly arises from preexisting PA (ie, SDC ex-PA). Morphologic evidence of a preexisting PA includes the finding of characteristic PA with chondromyxoid stroma or the presence of a hyalinized nodule (**Fig. 4**A–C).

Prior estimates suggest that approximately 50% of SDCs are ex-PA based on patient history and morphology[5,7,19,20]; however, more recent data incorporating cytogenetic changes estimate that up to 80% of SDCs are ex-PA.[21]

Whenever the diagnosis of carcinoma ex-PA is made, several important tumor features should be documented because they predict prognosis

Fig. 3. (continued). C) Sarcomatoid SDC showing an area with high-grade malignant spindle cells in a somewhat fascicular growth pattern. Most of this tumor was sarcomatoid, but scattered areas adjacent to the main tumor showed more conventional SDC confirming the diagnosis (both H&E, original magnification ×100). (*D*) Oncocytic SDC showing tumor cells with abundant oncocytic cytoplasm and occasional prominent nucleoli infiltrating adjacent salivary gland and soft tissue (H&E, original magnification ×200).

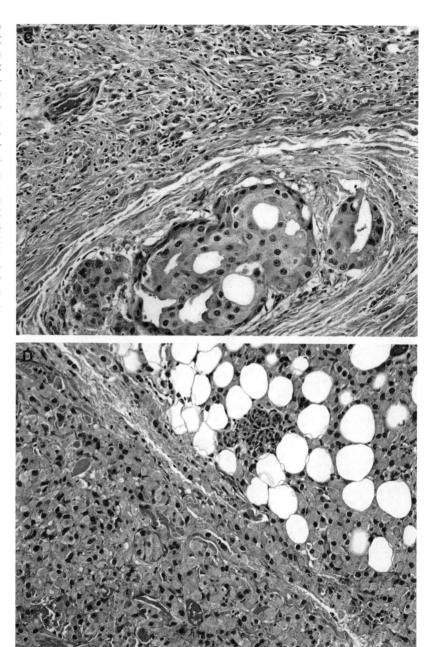

and can influence management. The type and/or grade of carcinoma is important because SDC ex-PA and other high-grade carcinomas ex-PA behave more aggressively than low-grade carcinoma ex-PA (eg, epithelial-myoepithelial carcinoma and myoepithelial carcinoma). Extent of invasion beyond the PA capsule is a second important feature because carcinoma ex-PA confined to the capsule or with minimal invasion are reported to be indolent, with most cured by excision. The recent fourth edition of the WHO classification expanded the definition of minimally invasive carcinoma ex-PA to include tumors with less than 4 to 6 mm of invasion beyond the PA capsule (this was previously defined as <1.5 mm).[22] However, limited literature specifically examines extent of invasion in the setting of SDC ex-PA, but at least 1 report found aggressive

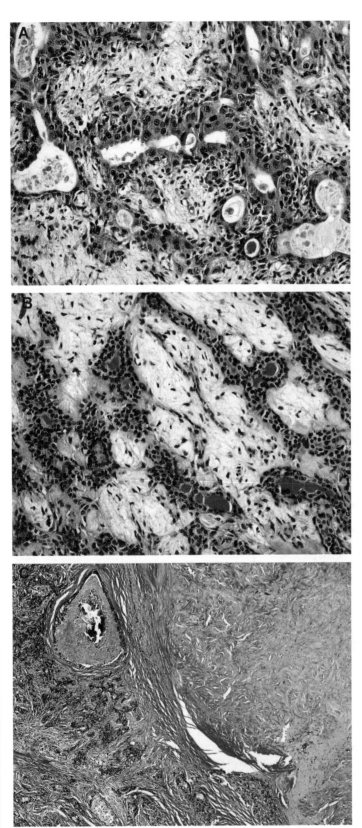

Fig. 4. SDC ex-PA. (*A*) SDC ex-PA showing an area of SDC within the stroma of a preexisting pleomorphic adenoma. The high-grade ductal cells are surrounding by smaller myoepithelial cells in this in situ example, and the surrounding chondromyxoid stroma is characteristic of PA (H&E, original magnification ×200). (*B*) Nearby area of the same tumor showing benign ductal cells of the preexisting PA (H&E, original magnification ×200). (*C*) Invasive SDC ex-PA with the invasive high-grade carcinoma seen on the left. The right side shows a hyalinized nodule, which is strong morphologic evidence of a preexisting PA (H&E, original magnification ×40).

features in 3 cases of SDC ex-PA with 2 mm or less invasion.[20]

A definitive prognostic significance of SDC ex-PA versus de novo SDC has not been shown, with the literature showing mixed results.[19,23] Evidence suggests that SDC arising in the setting of recurrent PA may be more aggressive with a worse prognosis than SDC ex-PA diagnosed at the initial diagnosis of PA.[23]

IMMUNOHISTOCHEMISTRY

SDC is generally positive for epithelial markers, such as epithelial membrane antigen,[7] AE1/AE3,[7] and CK7.[13,17] CK5/6 and p63 are rarely positive[13,24] but can be positive in those rare examples with squamous differentiation. CK20 is usually negative. Breast markers GATA3,[13] mammaglobin,[25] and gross cystic disease fluid protein 15 (GCDFP-15)[7] are commonly positive. Rare cases of S100 positivity have been described in the literature, but S100 is usually negative, as are most specific myoepithelial markers (SMAs; calponin, and so forth).[7,13] Hormone receptor expression widely varies depending on the study; however, AR expression is common in SDC (69% to >95%), reflective of the apocrine phenotype (Fig. 5).[9,11,13,24] Expression of estrogen receptor (ER) is rare and progesterone receptor (PR) positivity is uncommon.[9] The rate of HER2 overexpression varies widely in the literature (15% to 43%) because of differences in grading methodologies and techniques.[24,26]

DIFFERENTIAL DIAGNOSIS

The diagnosis of SDC is based on the finding of a high-grade primary salivary gland adenocarcinoma showing apocrine differentiation. Difficulty may be encountered in patients with variant morphology, and ample sampling of the tumor may be helpful to find areas of classic features. An in situ component or prior PA (by morphology or history) can be helpful to confirm a primary salivary tumor. AR positivity by IHC is found in most cases but should be used with the understanding that a variety of other primary salivary gland tumors and metastases may show AR expression.

MUCOEPIDERMOID CARCINOMA

SDC and high-grade MEC may show some morphologic overlap. MECs classically have 3 cell populations of epidermoid, intermediate, and goblet cells/mucocytes, whereas these various cell types are not common in SDC. Overt squamous and mucinous differentiation are uncommon in SDC and typically are only seen in variants, as discussed earlier.[7,9] The absence of epidermoid and mucous cells argues against high-grade MEC,[9] whereas cribriform architecture favors SDC.[7] Immunohistochemically, p63 is positive in MEC and usually negative in SDC.[2] Most SDCs are positive for AR, whereas this is seen in only a small subset (~5%) of MECs. In more challenging cases, fluorescence in situ hybridization (FISH) for MAML2 may be useful because at least half of high-grade MECs are positive for the *MECT1-MAML2* rearrangement.

ONCOCYTIC CARCINOMA

The abundant eosinophilic cytoplasm of SDC can also raise consideration for oncocytic carcinoma. Oncocytic carcinoma is much rarer than SDC, and SDC should be excluded when a tumor is suggestive of a high-grade oncocytic carcinoma. Oncocytic carcinoma shows tumor cells with abundant finely granular cytoplasm caused by numerous mitochondria. IHC for cytochrome-c oxidase or special stains for phosphotungstic acid hematoxylin can confirm the abundance of mitochondria, but this is not specific because various tumors can have true oncocytic change.[6,7,9] Oncocytic carcinoma typically has solid organoid to trabecular growth and can show high-grade nuclear features. In contrast with SDC, comedonecrosis is not common. The most important distinguishing feature between SDC and oncocytic carcinoma is the identification of apocrine differentiation in SDC. Areas with apocrine differentiation may be hard to find in oncocytic variant SDC, requiring additional sampling for histology. IHC for AR, Her2neu, and GATA3 might be helpful because these are more likely to be positive in SDC.[2] Importantly, such IHC should be performed in areas with the most morphologically apparent apocrine differentiation.

ACINIC CELL CARCINOMA

AciCC is defined as having serous acinar differentiation indicated by basophilic cytoplasmic zymogen granules.[2] AciCC is commonly low grade but, because of the abundant cytoplasm, may enter the differential diagnosis with SDC. In most cases, AciCC lacks the nuclear pleomorphism, increased mitotic activity, and necrosis commonly found in SDC.[7] High-grade transformation (HGT) can occur in AciCC, but, in most patients, these areas of HGT have a basaloid appearance. In most patients, thorough examination identifies areas of typical AciCC. In more challenging cases, IHC may be helpful in that SOX10 and DOG1 are

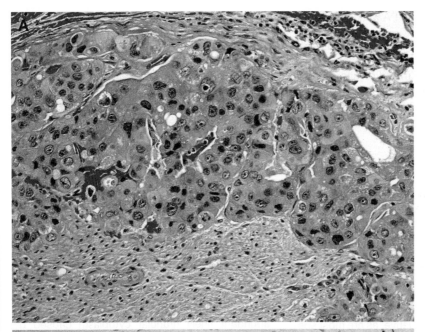

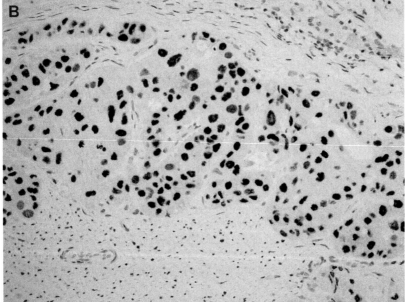

Fig. 5. Androgen receptor expression in SDC. (*A*) This focus of perineural SDC shows classic morphologic features with abundant finely granular to vacuolated cytoplasm and considerable nuclear enlargement and pleomorphism (H&E, original magnification ×200). (*B*) Androgen receptor expression can be variable in SDC but is strong and fairly diffuse in this example (androgen receptor, original magnification ×200).

commonly coexpressed in AciCC but are negative in SDC.[27]

INTRADUCTAL CARCINOMA (FORMERLY LOW-GRADE CRIBRIFORM Cystadenocarcinoma/Low-GRADE SALIVARY DUCT CARCINOMA)

This entity has undergone several nomenclature revisions, with the recent WHO classification of head and neck tumors using the term intraductal carcinoma.[8,28] This tumor is an intraductal proliferation of neoplastic cells surrounded by a myoepithelial cell layer, similar to DCIS of breast.[8,28] Intraductal carcinoma can be low, intermediate, or high grade, with high-grade forms entering the differential diagnosis with SDC. Classic intercalated duct–like intraductal carcinoma is S100 and SOX10 positive and AR negative, but an apocrine variant exists that is S100 and SOX10 negative and AR positive. Such cases of high-grade apocrine intraductal carcinoma are distinguished from SDC by the presence of a surrounding myoepithelial cell layer highlighted by p40/p63 or SMA.[6,28] This apocrine variant of intraductal carcinoma may represent a precursor lesion to more widely invasive SDC because there are also some genetic similarities.[28] Small areas of invasion may be seen in tumors classifiable as intraductal carcinoma, but the significance of this remains to be determined and intraductal carcinomas are generally indolent with an excellent prognosis after complete excision.[8,28] The distinction between intraductal carcinoma and SDC is important to avoid overtreatment.

OTHER SALIVARY GLAND NEOPLASMS WITH HIGH-GRADE TRANSFORMATION

A variety of otherwise low-grade salivary gland neoplasms (AciCC, myoepithelial carcinoma, adenoid cystic carcinoma, and epithelial-myoepithelial carcinoma) can undergo HGT with areas of cribriform architecture and/or comedonecrosis.[6] In such patients, it is helpful to identify areas of the conventional lower-grade tumor that can be aided by IHC.[6,11] This point is critical to note because some cases of SDC are AR negative/nonapocrine, and, as such, HGT of other malignancies must be excluded. Thorough gross sectioning and sampling is recommended.[6] In general, tumors with HGT are more basaloid than typical SDC.

METASTATIC CARCINOMA

A common differential diagnostic consideration in cases of SDC is metastatic carcinoma, including both head and neck and more distant primaries. Specifically, metastatic squamous cell carcinoma (SqCC) arising in the head and neck (particularly cutaneous primaries) can metastasizes to intraparotid/periparotid lymph nodes. The abundant eosinophilic cytoplasm in nonkeratinizing SqCC closely mimics that of SDC. However, IHC for AR and p63/p40 can be helpful.[6,11,13] Caution is needed in the use of GATA3 for this distinction because many cutaneous and some mucosal SqCCs are GATA3 positive.[29] Even with the combined use of morphology and IHC, rare cases of SDC with extensive squamous differentiation can be challenging to distinguish, with clinical correlation and extensive sampling being helpful. Primary SqCC of the parotid gland is exceedingly rare.[11]

Metastatic disease from more distant sites below the clavicles are rare but should also be considered in the setting of a high grade adenocarcinoma in the parotid gland. While breast carcinoma only rarely accounts for distant metastases to intraparotid lymph nodes, the extensive morphologic overlap of these entities may lead to this consideration.[30] In rare instances, an apocrine subtype of mammary carcinoma recapitulates morphologic and immunohistochemical findings in SDC, and, as such, additional clinical and radiographic correlation would be required to make the distinction. ER and PR expression is rare in SDC and therefore favors metastatic breast carcinoma.[2] Likewise, prostatic carcinoma can be immunophenotypically similar to SDC with expression of AR and prostatic acid phosphatase (up to 50% of SDCs).[5] In cases in which a metastasis is included in the differential diagnosis, an in situ component or preexisting PA favors a salivary gland primary.[7]

PROGNOSIS AND TREATMENT

SDC is an aggressive malignancy. In a 20-year review of SDC, two-thirds of patients presented with advanced (T3/T4) disease and 54% had cervical lymph node metastases.[19] Local recurrences occurred in 48%. Decreased survival is significantly correlated with clinical stage IV disease, nodal status, positive surgical margins, extranodal extension, and perineural invasion.[31] Lymph node metastasis is a strong predictor of death from disease, with only 19% of node-positive patients alive and free of disease at 5 years.[13] Fifty-two percent of patients died of disease or developed incurable recurrences at a median follow-up of 23 months. Current treatment of SDC reflects this aggressive behavior in that most patients undergo surgical resection, lymph node dissection, and adjuvant radiotherapy. Chemotherapy is also added for some patients. An exception to this aggressive therapy may be possible in at least some patients with encapsulated/in situ SDC ex-PA and possibly those with minimally invasive SDC ex-PA, but at least close follow-up should be recommended for these patients.

EMERGING THERAPIES

Because of the aggressive nature of SDC and the presence of metastatic disease in many patients, there is considerable investigation into the possibility of systemic therapies. Several therapeutic and prognostic markers have been investigated.

Given the high rate of AR expression, the possible utility of androgen deprivation therapy (ADT) for SDC was proposed as early as 2000.[5,32,33] Only limited studies are available but at least some cases seem to show a benefit from the addition of ADT.[34–36] Prostatic adenocarcinoma, another tumor with AR, has shown promise

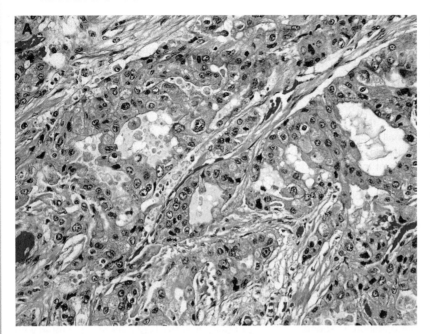

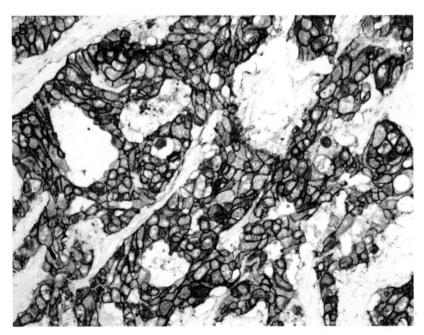

Fig. 6. Her2 expression is common SDC with strong (3+) staining, as seen in this case correlating well with amplification by FISH (*A*, H&E, original magnification ×200; *B*, Her2, immunohistochemistry, original magnification ×200).

with the use of ADT.[37] However, ADT resistance has been shown to occur because of expression of an AR splice site variant, AR-V7. This variant form causes resistance through loss of the androgen-binding domain but maintenance of the DNA-binding function.[38] AR-V7 is also expressed in some cases of SDC and may represent a source of ADT resistance in this disease as well.[16,32] Further investigation is needed regarding the use of ADT in SDC.

Targeting of *ERRB2* amplification with Her2/neu blockade is another avenue that is being pursued in treatment of SDC. Similar to breast cancer, HER2/neu overexpression as a result of this amplification is common and is seen in approximately one-quarter to one-third of all SDCs.[16,39,40] The most appropriate method for determining *ERBB2* amplification in SDC is not as well established as in breast cancer. Some institutions report a combination of HER2/neu IHC (**Fig. 6**) and FISH, whereas others use FISH only. Studies reporting both IHC and FISH results indicate good correlation between these methodologies.[39,40] Clinical trials to assess the response to trastuzumab are not available but limited small series and case reports show some evidence of possible modest successes through the addition of this agent.[3,41–43]

Programmed death-ligand 1 (PD-L1) expression has been identified in a small subset of SDC (22%–26%). There is conflicting information regarding its role as a prognostic and therapeutic marker; however, there are currently a limited number of studies examining this target for immune therapy.[44–46]

Molecular characterization of SDC via whole-exome sequencing, RNA sequencing, and immunohistochemical analyses found a high mutational burden compared with other salivary gland tumors.[16] TP53 mutations were the most common finding (55%) and were associated with more aggressive behavior (higher rates of recurrence and metastases).[16] Sixty-one percent of SDCs were found to harbor potentially targetable molecular alterations.

The phosphatidylinositol 3 kinase (PI3K) pathway, including mutations of PIK3CA and phosphatase and tensin homolog (PTEN) loss, have been proposed as potential therapeutic targets in SDC. The PI3K pathway is associated with critical cellular functions and a variety of molecular inhibitors are available at various steps in this pathway (eg, mammalian target of rapamycin [mTOR] inhibitors). The loss of PTEN expression is variably reported in the literature, between 28% and 50%, which may be associated with alterations in the PI3K pathway.[24,47] Similarly, activating mutation in PIK3CA have been reported in approximately a quarter of SDCs.[48,49] Interestingly, overexpression of HER2 has been found to be associated with reciprocal alterations along the PI3K pathway, suggesting the potential importance of evaluating multiple pathways and alterations in cases of SDC.

A variety of other less common molecular alterations have been reported, and some of these may represent useful therapeutic targets. Genomic alterations in the BRAF gene are reported not to occur, or to only rarely occur in SDC,[13,40,50] and experience with BRAF V600E targeted therapy is limited to only a case report of SDC with osseous metastases. A combination of dabrafenib (BRAF inhibitor) and trametinib (mitogen-activated protein kinase [MEK] inhibitor) showed improvement to the metastatic deposits. This regimen was discontinued and palliative radiotherapy was initiated after a restaging PET/computed tomography scan after 13 months showed multiple new metastases.[51] Further investigation is warranted to determine the utility of targeted therapy in this context.

High expression of EGFR has been found in SDC but the prognostic and treatment significance of this marker is unclear.[52] Expression of EGFR has been detected in 70% to 80% of SDCs, with approximately a quarter showing strong (3+) expression.[39,53] Gene amplification was not detected in any of these cases and mutations were rare. One study showed that EGFR expression was associated with a significantly better disease-free survival.[53]

SDCs lacking expression of ERβ have been correlated with increased local and regional recurrences. Downregulation is associated with adverse clinical features.[31] Therapeutic targeting of ERβ may useful in the management of SDC in some patients.

Because of the variety of molecular alterations and interplay of these pathways in SDC, comprehensive molecular characterization are likely to be important for selecting the best individualized therapy for patients with this aggressive malignancy.

SUMMARY

SDC is an aggressive malignancy associated with frequent metastases, local recurrence, and significant mortality. Many SDCs are associated with an antecedent PA and this remains of uncertain prognostic significance. The quintessential morphologic feature of SDC is apocrine differentiation in a high-grade adenocarcinoma. Perineural and lymphovascular invasion can often be identified. Several variant SDC morphologies have been described, which can make accurate diagnosis challenging, but thorough sampling and IHC can be helpful to achieve the correct diagnosis.

Because of the aggressive nature of this disease, current treatment is also aggressive and commonly includes excision with lymph node dissection, radiation, and chemotherapy, but a standardized treatment protocol does not exist. Continued investigation into prognostic and/or therapeutic markers such as ADT, HER2 blockade, BRAF, EGFR, ERβ, and PD-L1 is ongoing, and comprehensive molecular characterization may be useful in the future for selecting the most appropriate treatment of these patients.

CLINICS CARE POINTS

- SDC is an aggressive form of salivary gland malignancy.

- Most cases of SDC have an apocrine morphology and are immunophenotypically positive for AR.

- Several morphologic variants of this malignancy exist, which may be diagnostic pitfalls.

- AR and HER2/neu expression are common. Although other molecular alterations have been identified, their significance on prognosis and therapy warrants additional studies.

- Surgical resection with lymph node resection is commonly used followed with or without radiation therapy. Systemic therapy is used in metastatic cases, although a standardized therapy regimen does not yet exist.

DISCLOSURE

The authors have nothing to disclose.

REFERENCES

1. Kleinsasser O, Klein HJ, Hubner G. Speichelgang-carcinome. Arch Klin Exp Ohren Nasen Kehlkopfheilkd 1968;192(1):100–15.

2. Sekhri R, Ortanca I, Boals C, et al. Salivary duct carcinoma: a case report of oncocytic variant with possible treatment implications and review of literature. Pathol Res Pract 2019;215(10):152549.

3. Park JC, Ma TM, Rooper L, et al. Exceptional responses to pertuzumab, trastuzumab, and docetaxel in human epidermal growth factor receptor-2 high expressing salivary duct carcinomas. Head Neck 2018;40(12):E100–6.

4. Fan C-Y, Melhem MF, Hosal AS, et al. Expression of Androgen receptor, epidermal growth factor receptor, and transforming growth factor α in salivary duct carcinoma. Arch Otolaryngol Head Neck Surg 2001;127(9):1075.

5. Fan CY, Wang J, Barnes EL. Expression of androgen receptor and prostatic specific markers in salivary duct carcinoma: an immunohistochemical analysis of 13 cases and review of the literature. Am J Surg Pathol 2000;24(4):579–86.

6. Udager AM, Chiosea SI. Salivary duct carcinoma: an update on morphologic mimics and diagnostic use of androgen receptor immunohistochemistry. Head Neck Pathol 2017;11(3):288–94.

7. Lewis JE, McKinney BC, Weiland LH, et al. Salivary duct carcinoma. Clinicopathologic and immunohistochemical review of 26 cases. Cancer 1996;77(2):223–30.

8. IARC WHO Classification of Tumours N 9, El-Naggar AK, Chan JKC, Jennifer RG, et al. WHO classification of head and neck tumours. 4th edition. Lyon, France: IARC; 2017.

9. McHugh JB, Visscher DW, Barnes EL. Update on selected salivary gland neoplasms. Arch Pathol Lab Med 2009;133(11):1763–74.

10. Simpson RHW. Salivary duct carcinoma: new developments—morphological variants including pure in situ high grade lesions; proposed molecular classification. Head Neck Pathol 2013;7(S1):48–58.

11. Williams L, Thompson LDR, Seethala RR, et al. Salivary duct carcinoma: the predominance of apocrine morphology, prevalence of histologic variants, and androgen receptor expression. Am J Surg Pathol 2015;39(5):705–13.

12. Nagao T, Gaffey TA, Visscher DW, et al. Invasive micropapillary salivary duct carcinoma: a distinct histologic variant with biologic significance. Am J Surg Pathol 2004;28(3):319–26.

13. Luk PP, Weston JD, Yu B, et al. Salivary duct carcinoma: clinicopathologic features, morphologic spectrum, and somatic mutations. Head Neck 2016;38(Suppl 1):E1838–47.

14. Simpson RHW, Prasad AR, Lewis JE, et al. Mucin-rich variant of salivary duct carcinoma: a clinicopathologic and immunohistochemical study of four cases. Am J Surg Pathol 2003;27(8):1070–9.

15. Henley J, Summerlin D-J, Potter D, et al. Intraoral mucin-rich salivary duct carcinoma. Histopathology 2005;47(4):436–7.

16. Dalin MG, Watson PA, Ho AL, et al. Androgen receptor signaling in salivary gland cancer. Cancers (Basel) 2017;9(2). https://doi.org/10.3390/cancers9020017.

17. Nagao T, Gaffey TA, Serizawa H, et al. Sarcomatoid variant of salivary duct carcinoma: clinicopathologic and immunohistochemical study of eight cases with review of the literature. Am J Clin Pathol 2004;122(2):222–31.

18. Di Palma S, Simpson RHW, Marchiò C, et al. Salivary duct carcinomas can be classified into luminal androgen receptor-positive, HER2 and basal-like phenotypes. Histopathology 2012;61(4):629–43.

19. Gilbert MR, Sharma A, Schmitt NC, et al. A 20-year review of 75 cases of salivary duct carcinoma. JAMA Otolaryngol Head Neck Surg 2016;142(5):489–95.

20. Griffith CC, Thompson LDR, Assaad A, et al. Salivary duct carcinoma and the concept of early carcinoma ex pleomorphic adenoma. Histopathology 2014;65(6):854–60.

21. Chiosea SI, Thompson LDR, Weinreb I, et al. Subsets of salivary duct carcinoma defined by

morphologic evidence of pleomorphic adenoma, PLAG1 or HMGA2 rearrangements, and common genetic alterations. Cancer 2016;122(20):3136–44.

22. Barnes L, Eveson JW, Reichart P, et al. Pathology and genetics of head and neck tumours. 3rd edition. Geneva (Switzerland): IARC; 2005.

23. Stodulski D, Mikaszewski B, Majewska H, et al. Parotid salivary duct carcinoma: a single institution's 20-year experience. Eur Arch Otorhinolaryngol 2019;276(7):2031–8.

24. Liang L, Williams MD, Bell D. Expression of PTEN, androgen receptor, HER2/neu, Cytokeratin 5/6, Estrogen Receptor-Beta, HMGA2, and PLAG1 in salivary duct carcinoma. Head Neck Pathol 2019; 13(4):529–34.

25. Soares CD, de Lima Morais TM, Carlos R, et al. Immunohistochemical expression of mammaglobin in salivary duct carcinomas de novo and salivary duct carcinoma ex pleomorphic adenoma. Hum Pathol 2019. https://doi.org/10.1016/j.humpath.2019.08.001.

26. Griffith CC, Schmitt AC, Little JL, et al. New developments in salivary gland pathology: clinically useful ancillary testing and new potentially targetable molecular alterations. Arch Pathol Lab Med 2017; 141(3):381–95.

27. Zhu S, Schuerch C, Hunt J. Review and updates of immunohistochemistry in selected salivary gland and head and neck tumors. Arch Pathol Lab Med 2015;139(1):55–66.

28. Bishop JA, Gagan J, Krane JF, et al. Low-grade apocrine intraductal carcinoma: expanding the morphologic and molecular spectrum of an enigmatic salivary gland tumor. Head Neck Pathol 2020. https://doi.org/10.1007/s12105-020-01128-0.

29. Miettinen M, McCue PA, Sarlomo-Rikala M, et al. GATA3. Am J Surg Pathol 2014;38(1):13–22.

30. Ando K, Masumoto N, Sakamoto M, et al. Parotid Gland Metastasis of Breast Cancer: Case Report and Review of the Literature. Breast Care (Basel) 2011;6(6):471–3.

31. Williams MD, Roberts D, Blumenschein GR, et al. Differential expression of hormonal and growth factor receptors in salivary duct carcinomas: biologic significance and potential role in therapeutic stratification of patients. Am J Surg Pathol 2007;31(11): 1645–52.

32. Yang RK, Zhao P, Lu C, et al. Expression pattern of androgen receptor and AR-V7 in androgen-deprivation therapy-naïve salivary duct carcinomas. Hum Pathol 2019;84:173–82.

33. Boon E, van Boxtel W, Buter J, et al. Androgen deprivation therapy for androgen receptor-positive advanced salivary duct carcinoma: a nationwide case series of 35 patients in The Netherlands. Head Neck 2018;40(3):605–13.

34. Soper MS, Iganej S, Thompson LDR. Definitive treatment of androgen receptor-positive salivary duct carcinoma with androgen deprivation therapy and external beam radiotherapy. Head Neck 2014;36: E4–7.

35. Locati LD, Perrone F, Cortelazzi B, et al. Clinical activity of androgen deprivation therapy in patients with metastatic/relapsed androgen receptor-positive salivary gland cancers. Head Neck 2016;38(5):724–31.

36. Jaspers HCJ, Verbist BM, Schoffelen R, et al. Androgen receptor–positive salivary duct carcinoma: a disease entity with promising new treatment options. J Clin Oncol 2011;29(16):e473–6.

37. Singer EA, Golijanin DJ, Miyamoto H, et al. Androgen deprivation therapy for prostate cancer. Expert Opin Pharmacother 2008;9(2):211–28.

38. Antonarakis ES, Lu C, Wang H, et al. AR-V7 and resistance to enzalutamide and abiraterone in prostate cancer. N Engl J Med 2014;371(11): 1028–38.

39. Williams MD, Roberts DB, Kies MS, et al. Genetic and expression analysis of HER-2 and EGFR genes in salivary duct carcinoma: empirical and therapeutic significance. Clin Cancer Res 2010;16(8): 2266–74.

40. Nardi V, Sadow PM, Juric D, et al. Detection of novel actionable genetic changes in salivary duct carcinoma helps direct patient treatment. Clin Cancer Res 2013;19(2):480–90.

41. Gibo T, Sekiguchi N, Gomi D, et al. Targeted therapy with trastuzumab for epidermal growth factor receptor 2 (HER2)-positive advanced salivary duct carcinoma: a case report. Mol Clin Oncol 2019. https://doi.org/10.3892/mco.2019.1875.

42. Limaye SA, Posner MR, Krane JF, et al. Trastuzumab for the treatment of salivary duct carcinoma. Oncologist 2013;18(3):294–300.

43. Takahashi H, Tada Y, Saotome T, et al. Phase II trial of trastuzumab and docetaxel in patients with human epidermal growth factor receptor 2-positive salivary duct carcinoma. J Clin Oncol 2019;37(2): 125–34.

44. Hamza A, Roberts D, Su S, et al. PD-L1 expression by immunohistochemistry in salivary duct carcinoma. Ann Diagn Pathol 2019;40:49–52.

45. Sato F, Akiba J, Kawahara A, et al. The expression of programed death ligand-1 could be related with unfavorable prognosis in salivary duct carcinoma. J Oral Pathol Med 2018;47(7):683–90.

46. Mukaigawa T, Hayashi R, Hashimoto K, et al. Programmed death ligand-1 expression is associated with poor disease free survival in salivary gland carcinomas. J Surg Oncol 2016;114(1):36–43.

47. Griffith CC, Seethala RR, Luvison A, et al. PIK3CA mutations and PTEN loss in salivary duct carcinomas. Am J Surg Pathol 2013;37(8):1201–7.

48. Dalin MG, Desrichard A, Katabi N, et al. Comprehensive molecular characterization of salivary duct carcinoma reveals actionable targets and similarity to apocrine breast cancer. Clin Cancer Res 2016; 22(18):4623–33.

49. Dogan S, Ng CKY, Xu B, et al. The repertoire of genetic alterations in salivary duct carcinoma including a novel HNRNPH3-ALK rearrangement. Hum Pathol 2019;88:66–77.

50. Ross JS, Gay LM, Wang K, et al. Comprehensive genomic profiles of metastatic and relapsed salivary gland carcinomas are associated with tumor type and reveal new routes to targeted therapies. Ann Oncol 2017;28(10):2539–46.

51. Lin VTG, Nabell LM, Spencer SA, et al. First-line treatment of widely metastatic BRAF -mutated salivary duct carcinoma with combined BRAF and MEK inhibition. J Natl Compr Canc Netw 2018; 16(10):1166–70.

52. Schmitt NC, Kang H, Sharma A. Salivary duct carcinoma: an aggressive salivary gland malignancy with opportunities for targeted therapy. Oral Oncol 2017; 74:40–8.

53. Masubuchi T, Tada Y, Maruya S, et al. Clinicopathological significance of androgen receptor, HER2, Ki-67 and EGFR expressions in salivary duct carcinoma. Int J Clin Oncol 2015;20(1):35–44.

Polymorphous Adenocarcinoma

Nora Katabi, MD, Bin Xu, MD, PhD*

KEYWORDS

- Polymorphous adenocarcinoma • Cribriform adenocarcinoma
- Cribriform adenocarcinoma of salivary gland • PRKD

Key points

- Polymorphous adenocarcinoma (PAC) is characterized with cytologic uniformity, architectural diversity, and frequent *PRKD1* hotspot mutations.

- Cribriform adenocarcinoma of salivary gland (CASG) is a tumor with lobulated growth pattern, predominant solid/microcystic/cribriform architecture, peripheral palisading, glomeruloid structures, and high frequency of *PRKD1, PRKD2*, or *PRKD3* fusion.

- PAC and CASG may represent tumors in the same morphologic spectrum; however, some pathologists regard them as 2 separate entities.

- Although PAC and CASG commonly affect minor salivary glands, they may occur in major salivary glands.

- Tumors with greater than or equal to 30% cribriform or greater than or equal to 10% papillary architectural patterns are associated with decreased disease-free survival.

ABSTRACT

Polymorphous adenocarcinoma (PAC) is typically originated from the minor salivary glands and is characterized by cytology uniformity and architectural diversity. PAC commonly harbors *PRKD1* E710D mutation. PAC has an excellent prognosis. However, greater than or equal to 10% papillary or greater than or equal to 30% cribriform pattern is an independent adverse prognostic factor. Cribriform adenocarcinoma of salivary gland (CASG) is a controversial entity that is considered within the same histologic spectrum of PAC in current classification schemes; however, it is regarded by some pathologists as a separate entity. CASG shows a propensity to base of tongue location, a lobulated growth pattern, a predominant solid/cribriform architecture, and a high frequency of *PRKD1/2/3* fusion.

OVERVIEW

Polymorphous adenocarcinoma (PAC) is defined by the World Health Organization (WHO) classification[1] as an infiltrative salivary gland carcinoma that is characterized by architectural diversity and cytologic uniformity. PAC is composed of a single type of uniform tumor cells that exhibit clear chromatin and inconspicuous nucleoli, resembling the nuclei of papillary thyroid carcinoma. The term "polymorphous" describes the various architectural patterns that may be seen in PAC.

Department of Pathology, Memorial Sloan Kettering Cancer Center, 1275 York Avenue, New York, NY 10065, USA
* Corresponding author.
E-mail address: xub@mskcc.org
Twitter: @binxu16 (B.X.)

Surgical Pathology 14 (2021) 127–136
https://doi.org/10.1016/j.path.2020.09.011

surgpath.theclinics.com

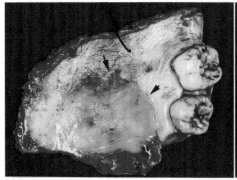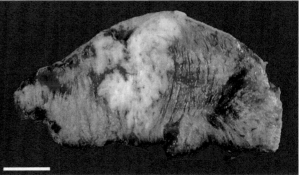

Fig. 1. Macroscopic appearance of polymorphous adenocarcinoma (PAC). (*Left*) A palate PAC is present as an indurated and bulging submucosal nodule (*arrows*) without direct surface involvement. (*Right*) Cross-section of a PAC/cribriform adenocarcinoma (CASG) originated from base of tongue shows an infiltrative multilobulated firm beige mass. Scale bar: 1 cm.

Approximately 95% of PAC affects the minor salivary glands of upper aerodigestive tract, most commonly the palate (in approximately 60% of cases, range: 49%–87%).[2–11] Other possible sites of origin include base of tongue, buccal mucosa, floor of mouth, lip, lateral tongue, retromolar trigone, sinonasal tract, oropharynx, and nasopharynx.[2–10] PAC may occasionally occur in major salivary glands, in particular the parotid gland, in approximately 3% (range: 0%–9%) of cases.[2–10]

Clinically, PAC occurs more frequently in women with a reported female to male ratio of approximately 2:1 (range: 1.3:1–2.15:1).[2–10] PAC may occur in a wide age range from 16 to 94 years, with a mean age of diagnosis in the 60s.[2–10]

GROSS FEATURES

Macroscopically, PAC typically presents as a submucosal nodule with or without surface ulceration. The tumor cross-section manifests as an unencapsulated, multilobulated, firm, beige to tan mass with lobulated or infiltrative borders (**Fig. 1**).

MICROSCOPIC FEATURES

At low power, PAC typically presents as an infiltrative unencapsulated mass (**Fig. 2**). The key diagnostic histologic features of PAC are its cytologic uniformity and architectural diversity. Architectural patterns that may be variably present include single filing in which tumor cells aligned as single columns resembling lobular carcinoma of breast; tubules; elongated trabeculae; solid nests; anastomosing reticular or microcystic structures; papillary projection with or without fibrovascular cores; and cribriform structures. The extracellular matrix can be myxoid and/or hyalinized. Targetoid arrangement of tubules and trabeculae around nerves and vessels and streaming of tumor cells

as single rows along nerve bundles are common histologic findings. Perineural invasion is frequent in PAC, being seen in 60% to 75% of cases.[3,12] Regardless of the architectural pattern, PAC is typically composed of one type of monotonous tumor cells that are characterized by open chromatin, and inconspicuous nucleoli, resembling the nuclei of papillary thyroid carcinoma (**Box 1**).

Of note, certain histologic features, although infrequent, may be identified (usually focally) in PAC, and the presence of these features does not exclude the diagnosis of PAC. These features include oncocytic changes, clear cell changes, mucocytes, foamy cells/sebaceous differentiation, coarse calcification, psammoma bodies, prominent myxoid stroma, and tumor necrosis (**Fig. 3**). Metaplastic changes such as oncocytic or clear cell alterations can occasionally give the false impression that there are 2 cell types within the tumor.

High-grade transformation is a rare phenomenon that has been reported in PAC. It is characterized by marked nuclear atypia, prominent nucleoli, high mitotic count, and tumor necrosis.[13,14]

ANCILLARY STUDIES, DIAGNOSTIC

IMMUNOHISTOCHEMISTRY

Typically, PAC is diffusely and strongly positive for S100,[10,15–17] SOX10,[18] CAM 5.2,[10,12] and CK7.[10] Focal immunoexpression of myoepithelial markers, for example, smooth muscle actin (SMA), muscle-specific actin (MSA), and glial fibrillary acidic protein (GFAP), can be seen in PAC.[10,16,17] The Ki-67 proliferation index is typically low (less than 10%).[3,10,12] However, elevated Ki-67 index may be seen in 10% to 20% of cases.[3,10,12]

Recently, several studies have reported that PAC usually has a p63-positive/p40-negative

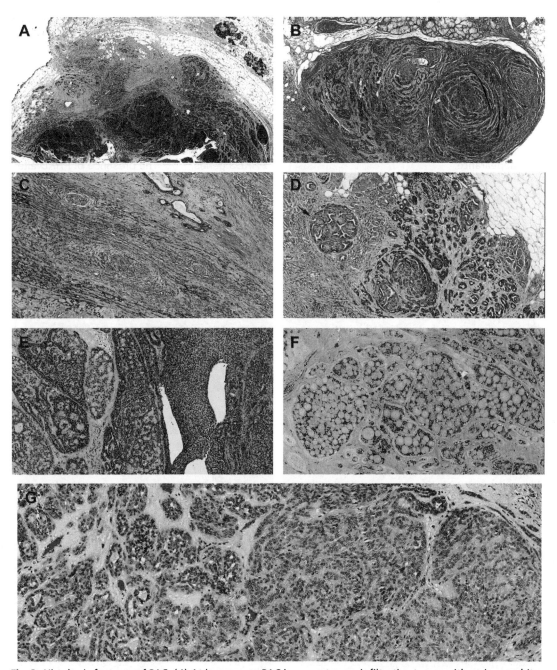

Fig. 2. Histologic features of PAC. (*A*) At low power, PAC is present as an infiltrative tumor with various architectural patterns. Streaming of tubules and nests may be evident at the periphery. (*B, C*) Perineural invasion with tumor cells arranged as single rows, tubules, and trabecular streaming around and between nerve bundles forming a targetoid appearance. Other architectural patterns that may be seen in PAC include papillary (*D, arrow*), tubules (*D, right*), trabecular-interlacing reticular (*E, left*), and solid (*E, right*), and cribriform pattern (*F*). (*G*) Regardless of the diverse architectural patterns, PAC is composed of one type of tumor cells typically with oval nuclei, pale fine chromatin, and inconspicuous nucleoli.

immunoprofile.[3,19,20] Notably, the p63 positivity is quite variable and can be focal/weak or diffuse and strong. Also important is the fact that the p63 staining pattern is typically diffuse or random, not biphasic, in contrast to some histologic mimickers (see differential diagnosis). It must also bee noted that the characteristic p63/p40 staining patterns seem to depend on laboratory conditions;

- PAC is characterized by cytologic uniformity
  and architectural diversity.
  - PAC is composed of a single type of tumor
    cells with pale nuclei.
  - PAC may contain multiple architectural
    patterns, which gives its polymorphous
    appearance.

occasional studies have not found this pattern to
be as consistent as others.[3,19]

MOLECULAR TESTING

In 2014, Weinreb and colleagues[21,22] were the first
to report the molecular signature of PAC. Most of
the PAC (73% - 89%) harbors *PRKD1* E710D hotspot mutation,[2,15,22,23] whereas 6% to 11%
contain fusions involving *PRKD1*, *PRKD2*, or
PRKD3 genes.[2,15,21] The presence of *PRKD* alterations is highly specific for PAC/cribriform adenocarcinoma of salivary gland (CASG, see the
following section) and has not been reported in

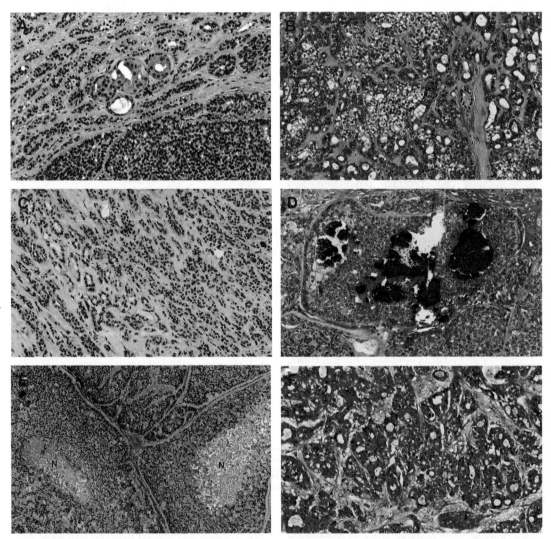

Fig. 3. Uncommon histologic features that may be seen in PAC. (*A*) Oncocytic changes (*blue arrow*). (*B*) Clear cell
changes. (*C*) Mucocytes (*green arrows*) and psammoma bodies (*red arrow*). (*D*) Coarse calcification and foamy/
sebaceous cells (*black arrow*). (*E*) Tumor necrosis (N). (*F*) Prominent myxoid stroma may be seen in a proportion
of PAC/CASG.

Table 1
Comparison between polymorphous adenocarcinoma and cribriform adenocarcinoma of salivary gland

	PAC	CASG
Primary site	Palate (49%–87%), MSG (13%–19%), BOT (0%–9%), major salivary gland (0%–9%)	BOT (24%–61%), MSG (26%–29%), palate (13%–57%), major salivary gland (0%–10%)
Growth pattern	Infiltrative, often with targetoid arrangement around nerves and vessels	Lobulated architecture separated by fibrous septa
Architecture	Highly variable, including single file arrangement, tubular, trabecular, reticular, solid, cribriform, and papillary	Relatively uniform, enriched in solid, microcystic, cribriform, and papillary growth
Cytologic features	One type of tumor cell with uniform pale open nuclei resembling papillary thyroid carcinoma	
Perineural invasion	Common (60%–75%)	Uncommon (38%)
Immunohistochemistry	Typically positive for S100, CK7, SOX10, and p63 Occasionally positive for GFAP, SMA, MSA, and EMA Typically negative for p40	
PRKD1 E710D hotspot mutation	73%–89%	0%–20%
PRKD1/2/3 fusion	6%–11%	70%–94%
Nodal metastasis at presentation	4%–6%	7%–100%

Note that a subset (25%–30%) of PAC/CASG spectrum shows indeterminate histologic features and may be difficult, if not impossible, to be classified as PAC or CASG.
Abbreviations: BOT, base of tongue/posterior tongue; MSG, minor salivary gland outside of palate and BOT.

other salivary gland neoplasms,[22,23] rendering it a useful molecular diagnostic tool for PAC.

CRIBRIFORM ADENOCARCINOMA OF SALIVARY GLAND

In 1999, Michal and colleagues[24] first coined the terminology "cribriform adenocarcinoma of the tongue" to describe a salivary gland carcinoma with a propensity to posterior tongue, lobulated architecture, a predominant solid, microcystic and cribriform growth pattern, and a uniform type of tumor cells with ground-glass optically cleared nuclei. Subsequent studies have shown that although cribriform adenocarcinoma most frequently occurs in posterior tongue/base of tongue, it may also affect palate, buccal mucosa, lip, tonsil, sinonasal tract, and rarely major salivary glands.[2,3,15,21,25–27] Therefore, a revised terminology of CASG has been suggested.

CASG shares certain histologic, immunophenotypic, and molecular similarity with PAC. A comparison between PAC and CASG is provided in **Table 1**. Histologically, both tumors are composed of one type of cells with pale optically cleared nuclei (**Fig. 4**). Unlike classic PAC, which usually shows an infiltrative growth and various architectural patterns, CASG tends to have lobulated growth separated by fibrous septa, and relatively uniform architecture predominantly composed of solid, microcystic, and/or cribriform patterns. Peripheral palisading and clefts, hemorrhage, and glomeruloid-like structures are common. The immunoprofile of CASG is indistinguishable from PAC.

Recently, it was reported that 75% to 94% of CASG harbor fusions involving *PRKD1*, *PRKD2*, or *PRKD3* genes,[2,15,21] with the fusion partners being *ARID1A* or *DDX3X*.[2,21] Although Weinreb and colleagues[22] only reported *PRKD* fusions in CASG, *PRKD1* E710D hotspot mutation is subsequently detected in a small subset (13%–20%) of CASG.[2,15]

In the initial series of 8 cases reported by Michal and colleagues, all patients had lymph node metastasis at presentation, which suggested a more aggressive clinical behavior of CASG. However, subsequent studies have reported a wide

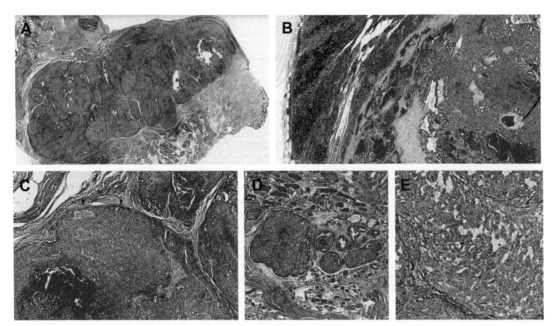

Fig. 4. Cribriform adenocarcinoma of salivary glands (CASG). (*A*) A CASG originated from base of tongue is composed of multiple tightly packed tumor nodules separated by fibrous septa. (*B*) The tumor is associated with nodal metastases at presentation. Arrowhead: papillary architecture is noted within the tumor. (*C*) CASG typically shows solid growth pattern with peripheral palisading (*black arrows*). Pools of blood ("blood lake") are a common histologic finding within the tumor. (*D*) CASG often has peripheral clefts within the tumor nests, giving the glomeruloid (G) appearance. (*E*) Microcystic architecture is common. The tumor is composed of a single type of tumor cells with optically clear nuclei.

range of frequency of nodal metastasis at presentation from 7% to 65%.[3,27,28] The great variation of nodal metastasis frequency reported in CASG may in part be attributed to the rarity of this tumor and the capability of a pathologist to recognize these tumors. A recent study has shown that only a fair interobserver agreement is achieved among expert head and neck pathologists in diagnosing CASG.[15] Nevertheless, the risk of nodal metastasis in CASG seems to be overall higher compared with 4% to 6% risk observed in patients with PAC.[3,7,10,11]

Interestingly, tumors with *PRKD* fusion, regardless of the histologic classification of PAC or CASG, are associated with a 50% initial risk of lymph node metastasis compared with 0% risk in tumors with *PRKD1* mutation.[2] Therefore, in challenging cases that are difficult to be further classified as PAC or CASG, molecular testing for *PRKD* genes may provide additional prognostic information in term of risk of nodal metastasis. On the other hand, the high rate of metastasis may also be partly a function of the frequent oropharyngeal location of CASG. It is well established that squamous cell carcinomas of the oropharynx frequently metastasize to cervical lymph nodes due to the unique microanatomy of this location, and other salivary gland tumor types show a higher rate of regional metastases when arising in the oropharynx.[29]

Currently, CASG is considered as a variant of PAC by the WHO classification.[1] However, this is controversial as some investigators consider CASG and PAC as 2 separate entities given the differences in histologic features and underlying molecular alterations.[30] Recent data suggest that CASG and PAC may represent a morphologic spectrum of the same tumor. Although the classic cases of PAC and CASG can be distinguished histologically, there is a subset of 25% to 30% of cases showing indeterminate histologic features that are difficult, if not impossible, to be labeled definitively as either conventional PAC or CASG.[2,3,15,21] The interobserver agreement even among expert head and neck pathologists in further classifying these tumors are fair to moderate at most.[15] Taken together, the findings suggest that PAC/CASG may represent a spectrum with classic PAC and *PRKD1* hotspot mutation at one end, CASG and *PRKD* fusions at the other, and indeterminate neoplasms with overlapping histology and molecular alterations in the middle.

Table 2
Comparison between polymorphous adenocarcinoma and adenoid cystic carcinoma

	PAC	Adenoid Cystic Carcinoma
Primary site	Minor salivary gland: >90% • Palate: 49%–87% Major salivary gland: 0%–9%	Minor salivary gland: 61%–63% • Palate: 21%–26% Major salivary gland: 37%
Architecture	Highly variable Single filing arrangement, tubular, trabecular, reticular, solid, cribriform, and papillary	Variable Tubular, cribriform, and solid
Cell composition	Cytologic uniformity: one type of tumor cells only	Biphasic showing ductal (epithelial) and myoepithelial differentiation
Nuclear features	Pale nuclei and open chromatin	Dark angulated nuclei
Perineural invasion	Common: 60%–75%	Common: 88%
Immunohistochemistry	S100: diffuse and strong CK7: diffuse and strong p63 positive/p40 negative	S100: patchy, in myoepithelial or ductal cells CK7: patchy, predominantly in ductal cells p63 positive/p40 positive in myoepithelial cells only
Molecular profile	*PRKD1* E710D mutation: 73%–89% *PRKD1/2/3* fusion: 6%–11%	Fusion involving *MYB, MYBL1*, or *NFIB* genes, most common being *MYB-NFIB* fusion: 60%–90%
Outcome	Excellent 10-y DSS: 94%–99% Risk of distant metastasis: 0%–3%	Poor 5-y DSS: 55%–89% Risk of distant metastasis: 8%–46%

Abbreviation: DSS, disease-specific survival.

DIFFERENTIAL DIAGNOSIS

ADENOID CYSTIC CARCINOMA

Table 2 provides a comparison between adenoid cystic carcinoma and PAC. Similar to PAC, adenoid cystic carcinoma predominantly occurs in minor salivary glands.[31–34] Approximately 21% to 26% occur in the palate.[31–34] Histologically, unlike PAC/CASG that exhibits 1 cell type, adenoid cystic carcinoma is biphasic and is composed of 2 cell types: ductal (epithelial) and myoepithelial. This feature is particularly important to differentiate adenoid cystic carcinoma from CASG, as both may show a predominant cribriform pattern with myxoid stroma and perineural invasion. The myoepithelial cells of adenoid cystic carcinoma typically contain angulated dark nuclei, giving adenoid cystic carcinoma its basaloid appearance. Both PAC and adenoid cystic carcinoma are commonly infiltrative, display various architectural patterns, and may contain myxoid stroma and hyalinized globules. However, adenoid cystic carcinoma is characterized with tubular, cribriform, and solid growth patterns, whereas lacks other patterns that may be seen in PAC (eg, single filing arrangement, papillary architecture) and

seems less architecturally diverse. Given the biphasic nature of adenoid cystic carcinoma, the immunohistochemical profile is usually more variable, showing patchy rather than diffuse staining for S100 and CK7. Recent reports have shown that adenoid cystic carcinoma is commonly p63 (+)/p40 (+), compared with p63 (+)/p40 (−) that is observed in PAC.[19,20] Moreover, the pattern of p63 and p40 in adenoid cystic carcinoma is clearly biphasic, whereas p63 staining in PAC is haphazard. In challenging cases, molecular testing for *MYB, MYBL1*, or *NFIB* gene fusions may be of use as 60% to 90% of adenoid cystic carcinoma carries signature fusions, in particular t(6,9) *MYB-NFIB* fusion.[31,35,36] Clinically, adenoid cystic carcinoma is associated with a dismal long-term outcome, compared with an excellent prognosis of PAC.[31–34]

OTHER S100-POSITIVE SALIVARY GLAND NEOPLASMS

Because PAC is diffusely positive for S100, its differential diagnosis, especially in small biopsy materials, includes other S100-positive salivary gland neoplasms such as secretory carcinoma, myoepithelial carcinoma, and epithelial-myoepithelial carcinoma.

Myoepithelial carcinoma and PAC share certain histologic and immunophenotypic similarities. Both tumors are composed of one type of cells, contain myxoid stroma, and may be positive for S100 and myoepithelial markers, for example, GFAP, p63, SMA, and MSA. However, myoepithelial carcinoma typically shows expansile lobulated growth pattern and lacks the architectural diversity observed in PAC. Perineural invasion is uncommon in myoepithelial carcinoma.[37,38] Myoepithelial carcinomas that are positive for p63 are usually also positive for p40, in contrast to PAC, which is usually p63 positive but p40 negative. In challenging cases, molecular testing for *PRKD* alteration may serve as a useful ancillary diagnostic tool.

Epithelial myoepithelial carcinoma is not typically as infiltrative as PAC and is composed of ductal and myoepithelial cells instead of 1 cell type. Moreover, S100 is not diffuse and stains the myoepithelial component in epithelial myoepithelial carcinoma. Both p63 and p40 are positive in the myoepithelial cell component of epithelial myoepithelial carcinoma, resulting in a biphasic staining pattern.

Compared with PAC, secretory carcinoma more often shows microcystic and papillary-cystic architecture and does not commonly show cribriform or single cell patterns. Secretory carcinoma harbors *ETV6* fusions.[39,40] GATA3, mammaglobin, and CK7 can be positive in both PAC and secretory carcinoma.[10,18,41,42]

DIAGNOSIS

In typical cases, histology alone is sufficient for the diagnosis. A diagnosis of PAC can be rendered using the following 3 characteristics:

1. Typical histologic features of PAC characterized by architectural diversity and cytologic uniformity with pale nuclei and fine chromatin.
2. An immunoprofile of diffuse and strong S100 and CK7 positivity.
3. The presence of *PRKD* alterations, in particular *PRKD1* E710D hotspot mutation.

PROGNOSIS

PAC has an overall excellent prognosis with a 10-year disease specific survival of 94% to 99%[4,5,28] and a 10-year recurrence free survival of 83% to 88%.[4,28] Distant metastasis is rare in PAC but may occur in up to 3% of cases.[3,5] Histologic architecture with greater than or equal to 10%

papillary pattern or greater than or equal to 30% cribriform pattern has been shown to be an independent adverse prognostic factor associated with decreased disease-free survival.[3] As discussed earlier, CASG and *PRKD1/2/3* fusion are associated with an increased risk of lymph node metastasis.[2,24,27]

SUMMARY

PAC is a salivary gland carcinoma that often occurs in minor salivary gland location, in particular palate. It is characterized by cytologic uniformity, architectural diversity, an immunoprofile with S100 (+)/CK7 (+)/p63 (+)/p40 (−), *PRKD1* E710D hotspot mutation, and an excellent outcome. CASG shares histologic and immunohistochemical features with PAC and has a propensity to base of tongue location. CASG is characterized by lobulated growth pattern, predominant solid and cribriform architectures, high frequency of *PRKD* fusions, and an increased risk of nodal metastasis. Regardless of the diagnosis of PAC or CASG, tumors with greater than or equal to 10% of papillae or greater than or equal to 30% cribriform architecture associated with decreased disease-specific survival.

CLINICS CARE POINTS

- PAC has a propensity to minor salivary gland, in particular the palate. However, PAC may affect major salivary glands on occasion.
- Compared with biphasic salivary gland tumors, for example, adenoid cystic carcinoma, pleomorphic adenoma, and epithelial-myoepithelial carcinoma, PAC is composed of one type of tumor cells with pale nuclei.
- PAC is among 1 of the 3 salivary gland carcinomas exhibiting diffuse and strong S100 positivity and one cell type; the others are secretory carcinoma and myoepithelial carcinoma.
- The presence of focal uncommon features, for example, oncocytes, mucocytes, foamy cells/sebaceous differentiation, and calcification, does not exclude PAC.
- A typical case of CASG can be recognized by its lobulated growth pattern, predominant solid and cribriform architecture, peripheral clefting, and glomeruloid structure. Neck dissection may be considered, as CASG is associated with a relatively high frequency of nodal metastasis.

DISCLOSURE

The authors have nothing to disclose. Research reported in this publication was supported in part by the Cancer Center Support Grant of the National Institutes of Health/National Cancer Institute under award number P30CA008748. The content is solely the responsibility of the authors and does not necessarily represent the official views of the National Institutes of Health.

REFERENCES

1. El-Naggar AK, Chan JKC, Grandis JR, et al. World Health Organization Classification of Tumours: pathology and genetics of head and neck tumours. 4th edition. Lyon (France): International Agency for Research on Cancer (IARC); 2017.
2. Sebastiao APM, Xu B, Lozada JR, et al. Histologic spectrum of polymorphous adenocarcinoma of the salivary gland harbor genetic alterations affecting PRKD genes. Mod Pathol 2020;33(1):65–73.
3. Xu B, Aneja A, Ghossein R, et al. Predictors of Outcome in the Phenotypic Spectrum of Polymorphous Low-grade Adenocarcinoma (PLGA) and Cribriform Adenocarcinoma of Salivary Gland (CASG): A Retrospective Study of 69 Patients. Am J Surg Pathol 2016;40(11):1526–37.
4. Elhakim MT, Breinholt H, Godballe C, et al. Polymorphous low-grade adenocarcinoma: A Danish national study. Oral Oncol 2016;55:6–10.
5. Patel TD, Vazquez A, Marchiano E, et al. Polymorphous low-grade adenocarcinoma of the head and neck: A population-based study of 460 cases. Laryngoscope 2015;125(7):1644–9.
6. Seethala RR, Johnson JT, Barnes EL, et al. Polymorphous low-grade adenocarcinoma: the University of Pittsburgh experience. Arch Otolaryngol Head Neck Surg 2010;136(4):385–92.
7. Evans HL, Luna MA. Polymorphous low-grade adenocarcinoma: a study of 40 cases with long-term follow up and an evaluation of the importance of papillary areas. Am J Surg Pathol 2000;24(10):1319–28.
8. Evans HL, Batsakis JG. Polymorphous low-grade adenocarcinoma of minor salivary glands. A study of 14 cases of a distinctive neoplasm. Cancer 1984;53(4):935–42.
9. Vincent SD, Hammond HL, Finkelstein MW. Clinical and therapeutic features of polymorphous low-grade adenocarcinoma. Oral Surg Oral Med Oral Pathol 1994;77(1):41–7.
10. Castle JT, Thompson LD, Frommelt RA, et al. Polymorphous low grade adenocarcinoma: a clinicopathologic study of 164 cases. Cancer 1999;86(2):207–19.
11. Kimple AJ, Austin GK, Shah RN, et al. Polymorphous low-grade adenocarcinoma: a case series and determination of recurrence. Laryngoscope 2014;124(12):2714–9.
12. Perez-Ordonez B, Linkov I, Huvos AG. Polymorphous low-grade adenocarcinoma of minor salivary glands: a study of 17 cases with emphasis on cell differentiation. Histopathology 1998;32(6):521–9.
13. Simpson RH, Pereira EM, Ribeiro AC, et al. Polymorphous low-grade adenocarcinoma of the salivary glands with transformation to high-grade carcinoma. Histopathology 2002;41(3):250–9.
14. Pelkey TJ, Mills SE. Histologic transformation of polymorphous low-grade adenocarcinoma of salivary gland. Am J Clin Pathol 1999;111(6):785–91.
15. Xu B, Barbieri AL, Bishop JA, et al. Histologic Classification and Molecular Signature of Polymorphous Adenocarcinoma (PAC) and Cribriform Adenocarcinoma of Salivary Gland (CASG): An International Interobserver Study. Am J Surg Pathol 2020;44(4):545–52.
16. Gnepp DR, Chen JC, Warren C. Polymorphous low-grade adenocarcinoma of minor salivary gland. An immunohistochemical and clinicopathologic study. Am J Surg Pathol 1988;12(6):461–8.
17. Regezi JA, Zarbo RJ, Stewart JC, et al. Polymorphous low-grade adenocarcinoma of minor salivary gland. A comparative histologic and immunohistochemical study. Oral Surg Oral Med Oral Pathol 1991;71(4):469–75.
18. Adkins BD, Geromes A, Zhang LY, et al. SOX10 and GATA3 in Adenoid Cystic Carcinoma and Polymorphous Adenocarcinoma. Head Neck Pathol 2019;14(2):406–11.
19. Atiq A, Mushtaq S, Hassan U, et al. Utility of p63 and p40 in Distinguishing Polymorphous Adenocarcinoma and Adenoid Cystic Carcinoma. Asian Pac J Cancer Prev 2019;20(10):2917–21.
20. Rooper L, Sharma R, Bishop JA. Polymorphous low grade adenocarcinoma has a consistent p63+/p40- immunophenotype that helps distinguish it from adenoid cystic carcinoma and cellular pleomorphic adenoma. Head Neck Pathol 2015;9(1):79–84.
21. Weinreb I, Zhang L, Tirunagari LM, et al. Novel PRKD gene rearrangements and variant fusions in cribriform adenocarcinoma of salivary gland origin. Genes Chromosomes Cancer 2014;53(10):845–56.
22. Weinreb I, Piscuoglio S, Martelotto LG, et al. Hotspot activating PRKD1 somatic mutations in polymorphous low-grade adenocarcinomas of the salivary glands. Nat Genet 2014;46(11):1166–9.
23. Andreasen S, Melchior LC, Kiss K, et al. The PRKD1 E710D hotspot mutation is highly specific in separating polymorphous adenocarcinoma of the palate from adenoid cystic carcinoma and pleomorphic adenoma on FNA. Cancer Cytopathol 2018;126(4):275–81.
24. Michal M, Skalova A, Simpson RH, et al. Cribriform adenocarcinoma of the tongue: a hitherto

unrecognized type of adenocarcinoma characteristically occurring in the tongue. Histopathology 1999; 35(6):495–501.

25. Michal M, Kacerovska D, Kazakov DV. Cribriform adenocarcinoma of the tongue and minor salivary glands: a review. Head Neck Pathol 2013;7(Suppl 1):S3–11.

26. Laco J, Kamaradova K, Vitkova P, et al. Cribriform adenocarcinoma of minor salivary glands may express galectin-3, cytokeratin 19, and HBME-1 and contains polymorphisms of RET and H-RAS proto-oncogenes. Virchows Arch 2012;461(5):531–40.

27. Skalova A, Sima R, Kaspirkova-Nemcova J, et al. Cribriform adenocarcinoma of minor salivary gland origin principally affecting the tongue: characterization of new entity. Am J Surg Pathol 2011;35(8):1168–76.

28. Mimica X, Katabi N, McGill MR, et al. Polymorphous adenocarcinoma of salivary glands. Oral Oncol 2019;95:52–8.

29. Navale P, Rooper LM, Bishop JA, et al. Mucoepidermoid carcinoma of the oropharynx: a tumor type with a propensity for regional metastasis unrelated to histologic grade. Hum Pathol 2019;93:1–5.

30. Gnepp DR. Salivary gland tumor "wishes" to add to the next WHO Tumor Classification: sclerosing polycystic adenosis, mammary analogue secretory carcinoma, cribriform adenocarcinoma of the tongue and other sites, and mucinous variant of myoepithelioma. Head Neck Pathol 2014;8(1):42–9.

31. Xu B, Drill E, Ho A, et al. Predictors of Outcome in Adenoid Cystic Carcinoma of Salivary Glands: A Clinicopathologic Study With Correlation Between MYB Fusion and Protein Expression. Am J Surg Pathol 2017;41(10):1422–32.

32. Moran JJ, Becker SM, Brady LW, et al. Adenoid cystic carcinoma. A clinicopathological study. Cancer 1961;14:1235–50.

33. Spiro RH, Huvos AG, Strong EW. Adenoid cystic carcinoma of salivary origin. A clinicopathologic study of 242 cases. Am J Surg 1974;128(4):512–20.

34. Fordice J, Kershaw C, El-Naggar A, et al. Adenoid cystic carcinoma of the head and neck: predictors of morbidity and mortality. Arch Otolaryngol Head Neck Surg 1999;125(2):149–52.

35. Mitani Y, Li J, Rao PH, et al. Comprehensive analysis of the MYB-NFIB gene fusion in salivary adenoid cystic carcinoma: Incidence, variability, and clinicopathologic significance. Clin Cancer Res 2010; 16(19):4722–31.

36. Persson M, Andren Y, Mark J, et al. Recurrent fusion of MYB and NFIB transcription factor genes in carcinomas of the breast and head and neck. Proc Natl Acad Sci U S A 2009;106(44):18740–4.

37. Kong M, Drill EN, Morris L, et al. Prognostic factors in myoepithelial carcinoma of salivary glands: a clinicopathologic study of 48 cases. Am J Surg Pathol 2015;39(7):931–8.

38. Xu B, Mneimneh W, Torrence DE, et al. Misinterpreted Myoepithelial Carcinoma of Salivary Gland: A Challenging and Potentially Significant Pitfall. Am J Surg Pathol 2019;43(5):601–9.

39. Skalova A, Vanecek T, Sima R, et al. Mammary analogue secretory carcinoma of salivary glands, containing the ETV6-NTRK3 fusion gene: a hitherto undescribed salivary gland tumor entity. Am J Surg Pathol 2010;34(5):599–608.

40. Xu B, Haroon Al Rasheed MR, Antonescu CR, et al. Pan-Trk immunohistochemistry is a sensitive and specific ancillary tool for diagnosing secretory carcinoma of the salivary gland and detecting ETV6-NTRK3 fusion. Histopathology 2020; 76(3):375–82.

41. Schwartz LE, Begum S, Westra WH, et al. GATA3 immunohistochemical expression in salivary gland neoplasms. Head Neck Pathol 2013;7(4):311–5.

42. Bishop JA, Yonescu R, Batista D, et al. Utility of mammaglobin immunohistochemistry as a proxy marker for the ETV6-NTRK3 translocation in the diagnosis of salivary mammary analogue secretory carcinoma. Hum Pathol 2013;44(10):1982–8.

Emerging Entities in Salivary Pathology

A Practical Review of Sclerosing Microcystic Adenocarcinoma, Microsecretory Adenocarcinoma, and Secretory Myoepithelial Carcinoma

Lisa M. Rooper, MD[a,b],*

KEYWORDS

- Salivary gland carcinomas • Sclerosing microcystic adenocarcinoma
- Microsecretory adenocarcinoma • Secretory myoepithelial carcinoma • Immunohistochemistry
- Molecular diagnostics

Key points

- Sclerosing microcystic adenocarcinoma, a low-grade salivary carcinoma that is similar to microcystic adnexal carcinoma of the skin, is composed of a biphasic population of ductal and myoepithelial cells arranged into highly infiltrative tubules and cords and embedded in a dense collagenous stroma.

- Microsecretory adenocarcinoma, a newly described low-grade salivary carcinoma defined by a unique *MEF2C-SS18* fusion, demonstrates anastomosing microcysts and tubules lined by attenuated eosinophilic cells with prominent basophilic secretions and variable amounts of myxohyaline stroma.

- Secretory myoepithelial carcinoma, a recently recognized variant of myoepithelial carcinoma, is composed of large eosinophilic cells that have a signet ring appearance because of prominent intracellular mucin vacuoles but demonstrate immunohistochemical evidence of myoepithelial differentiation.

ABSTRACT

In recent years, increased molecular testing and improved immunohistochemical panels have facilitated more specific classification of salivary gland carcinomas, leading to recognition of several novel tumor types and unique histologic variants. Sclerosing microcystic adenocarcinoma, microsecretory adenocarcinoma, and secretory myoepithelial carcinoma are three such recently described entities that demonstrate low-grade cytology, production of prominent secretory material, and variable amounts of sclerotic stroma. This review provides a practical overview of these important and overlapping emerging entities in salivary gland pathology with a focus on distinctive histologic features and helpful ancillary studies that differentiate them from a wide range of familiar morphologic mimics.

OVERVIEW

In the last decade, the molecular underpinnings of most salivary gland carcinomas have been characterized in detail.[1–13] At the same time, immunohistochemical panels and mutation-specific antibodies have been developed that can also

---

[a] Department of Pathology, The Johns Hopkins University School of Medicine, Baltimore, MD, USA;
[b] Department of Oncology, The Johns Hopkins University School of Medicine, Baltimore, MD, USA
* Corresponding author. The Johns Hopkins Medical Institutions, 401 North Broadway, Weinberg 2242, Baltimore, MD 21231-2410.
E-mail address: rooper@jhmi.edu
Twitter: @LisaRooperMD (L.M.R.)

Surgical Pathology 14 (2021) 137–150
https://doi.org/10.1016/j.path.2020.10.003
1875-9181/21/© 2020 Elsevier Inc. All rights reserved.

surgpath.theclinics.com

reliably differentiate many salivary tumor types.[6,14–24] This enhanced ancillary testing has allowed for more precise classification of known salivary entities, not only facilitating correct diagnosis of individual tumors with unusual morphology but also fostering identification of novel histologic variants that were previously grouped into other categories. Furthermore, improved understanding of the morphologic boundaries of existing diagnoses has also crystallized recognition of small groups of tumors with unique characteristics that do not fit into conventional classifications and merit recognition as separate entities. Sclerosing microcystic adenocarcinoma (SMA), microsecretory adenocarcinoma (MSA), and secretory myoepithelial carcinoma (SMC) are three such emerging diagnoses that all demonstrate low-grade cytology, production of prominent secretory material, and variable amounts of sclerotic stroma. This review provides a practical overview of these important and overlapping emerging entities in salivary gland pathology with a focus on distinctive histologic features and helpful ancillary studies that can differentiate them from each other and from a wide range of more familiar morphologic mimics.

SCLEROSING MICROCYSTIC ADENOCARCINOMA

INTRODUCTION

SMA is a tumor of presumed salivary origin that is morphologically similar to microcystic adnexal carcinoma (MAC) of the skin. SMA was initially characterized as a unique head and neck mucosal entity by Mills and colleagues[25] in 2016, with eight cases reported in the literature under this name.[26,27] However, at least seven additional cases with identical morphology have previously been described in detail under other names including MAC, sclerosing sweat duct–like carcinoma, or syringomatous adenocarcinoma.[28–34] To date, SMA has exclusively been reported in minor salivary sites including the tongue, lip mucosa, floor of mouth, buccal mucosa, and nasopharynx. Although follow-up data are limited, patients with SMA have had uniformly good outcomes without locoregional recurrence or distant metastases.[25–27,29,30,32,33]

MICROSCOPIC FEATURES

Like its cutaneous counterpart MAC, SMA has a distinctive low-power appearance, with deeply infiltrative nests, cords, and tubules of tumor cells embedded in prominent desmoplastic to densely collagenous stroma (Fig. 1A). Indeed, the stroma of SMA can occupy more volume than the tumor epithelium. SMA is composed of a biphasic population of bland eosinophilic to clear cells, with a flattened rim of peripheral myoepithelial cells surrounding central cuboidal ductal cells (Fig. 1B). These ductal cells make lumens of various sizes containing occasional dense, globular eosinophilic secretory material. The nuclei are round to oval and monotonous with evenly dispersed chromatin and occasional nucleoli (Fig. 1C). Mitotic figures are not conspicuous. Perineural invasion is commonly seen (Fig. 1D).

IMMUNOHISTOCHEMISTRY

The biphasic nature of SMA (Fig. 2A) is evident on immunohistochemistry, with the central ductal component showing positivity for pancytokeratin and CK7 (Fig. 2B) and the peripheral myoepithelial cell population expressing smooth muscle actin, S100, p63 (Fig. 2C), and p40.[25–27] The luminal secretions are positive for mucicarmine (Fig. 2D).

MOLECULAR TESTING

The molecular underpinnings of SMA have not yet been well described. One case submitted for RNA-seq was negative for fusions.[35] A recent study of cutaneous MAC highlighted mutually exclusive *p53* and *JAK1* mutations,[36] but it is unclear whether SMA shares these alterations.

DIFFERENTIAL DIAGNOSIS

Although the histologic appearance of SMA is unique within the salivary spectrum, there are several tumors that can demonstrate overlapping morphology and immunophenotype. Perhaps the most significant mimic is squamous cell carcinoma (SCC), which also has dense eosinophilic cytoplasm and can grow in highly infiltrative nests and cords (Fig. 3A). Of course, the presence of overt keratinization or associated squamous dysplasia is not generally seen with SMA and confirms a diagnosis of SCC. Most cases of SCC that demonstrate predominantly cord-like architecture are high grade and also show significantly more cytologic atypia and prominent mitotic figures than SMA. The tubular variant of adenoid cystic carcinoma (ACC) is composed of a biphasic population of epithelial and myoepithelial cells that can show deeply infiltrative growth and stromal sclerosis that parallels SMA (Fig. 3B). However, ACC tends to have at least focally well-developed cribriform architecture and generally shows more pronounced cytologic atypia than SMA with hyperchromatic, angulated nuclei.

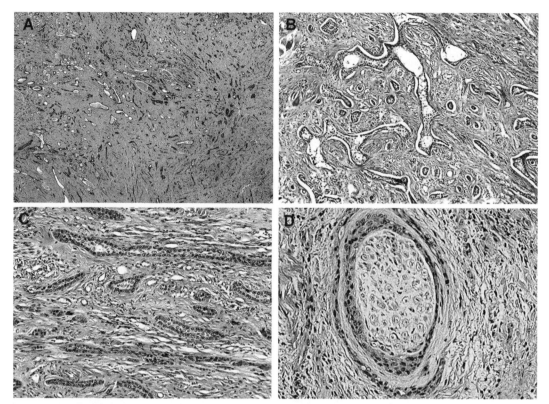

Fig. 1. SMA is highly infiltrative with prominent dense collagenous stroma (*A*, original magnification ×2). It is composed of nests, cords, and tubules, with scant eosinophilic secretory material (*B*, original magnification ×10). SMA contains a biphasic population of bland flattened to cuboidal eosinophilic cells, with distinct outer myoepithelial and inner ductal components (*C*, original magnification ×40). Perineural invasion is frequently seen (*D*, original magnification ×40). (*Courtesy of* J. Bishop, MD, Dallas, TX; and M.S. Hsieh, MD, PhD, Taipei, Taiwan.)

Detection of *MYB* or *MYBL1* rearrangements can also confirm the diagnosis of ACC in 50% to 80% of cases.[37–39] The eosinophilic cytoplasm, infiltrative and corded architecture, and prominent hyalinized stroma of SMA can also show some overlap with salivary clear cell carcinoma (CCC). In contrast to SMA, CCC is a monophasic neoplasm with diffuse positivity for p63 and p40 and negativity for other myoepithelial markers. CCC also harbor characteristic *EWSR1* rearrangements.[1] Mucoepidermoid carcinoma (MEC) can occasionally demonstrate a predominance of tubular growth and stromal sclerosis that mimics SMA (**Fig.** 3C). But although SMA shows scant intraluminal eosinophilic secretions, the presence of well-developed goblet cells and abundant mucin production favors classification as MEC. A diagnostic *MAML2* fusion is identified in 50% to 80% of MEC.[40–42] The classic form of polymorphous adenocarcinoma (PAC) also demonstrates predominantly tubular architecture and can occasionally be associated with abundant hyalinized

stroma (**Fig.** 3D). However, PAC is a monophasic tumor that is generally composed of columnar cells with more abundant cytoplasm than SMA. Identification of point mutations in *PRKD1* or rearrangements of *PRKD1, 2*, or *3* can confirm a diagnosis of PAC.[8,9]

SUMMARY

SMA is a unique tumor of presumed minor salivary origin that shows significant morphologic overlap with MAC of the skin. It demonstrates deeply infiltrative cords and tubules composed of cuboidal to flattened eosinophilic cells with bland round to oval nuclei embedded in dense sclerotic stroma. SMA contains a biphasic population of ductal cells that are strongly positive for AE1/AE3 and CK7 and myoepithelial cells that are positive for p63, p40, S100, smooth muscle actin, and calponin. SMA also produces scant eosinophilic globular luminal secretions that are positive for mucicarmine. Biphasic architecture, bland cytology, and lack of

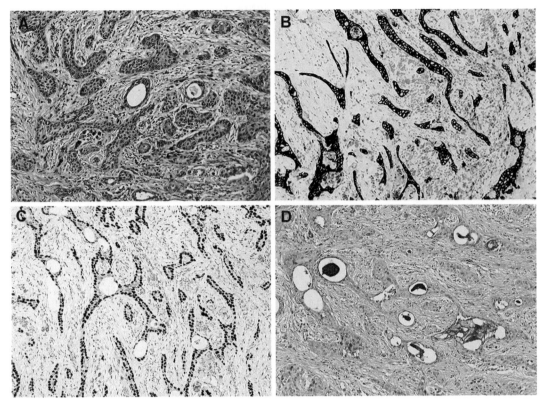

Fig. 2. Immunohistochemistry can highlight the biphasic nature of SMA (*A*, original magnification ×20) with CK7 strongly highlighting the central ductal cells (*B*, original magnification ×20) and p63 staining the abluminal myoepithelial cells (*C*, original magnification ×20). The globular eosinophilic intraluminal secretions are also positive for mucicarmine (*D*, original magnification ×20). (*Courtesy of* J. Bishop, MD, Dallas, TX; and M.S. Hsieh, MD, PhD, Taipei, Taiwan.)

keratinization are some of the most helpful features for differentiating SMA from mimics including SCC, ACC, CCC, MEC, and PAC.

MICROSECRETORY ADENOCARCINOMA

INTRODUCTION

MSA is a novel salivary gland tumor described by Bishop and colleagues[35] in 2019. It was identified among tumors that had previously been grouped in the heterogeneous adenocarcinoma not otherwise specified category. Although MSA was initially defined by recognition of recurrent *MEF2C-SS18* fusions, it also demonstrates distinctive histologic and immunohistochemical features that facilitate its diagnosis and further support classification as a unique pathologic entity. To date, five cases of MSA have been reported in the literature.[35] Most of these tumors have arisen in minor salivary gland sites, including the buccal mucosa and palate, but one case occurred in the parotid gland. Although minimal

data are available regarding the clinical course and prognosis of MSA, all reported cases have demonstrated a low-grade histologic appearance.

MICROSCOPIC FEATURES

MSA tends to be overall well-circumscribed but shows irregular borders with at least focally infiltrative growth into surrounding tissues (**Fig. 4**A). Tumors generally have a moderate amount of fibrous to myxohyaline stroma with areas of increased sclerosis at the center of the tumor (**Fig. 4**B). MSA is composed of a monophasic population of intercalated duct-like epithelioid cells with variable amounts of eosinophilic cytoplasm. These cells are predominantly arranged in anastomosing microcysts and tubules with flattened epithelial lining, but nests and cords of plumper cells can be interspersed throughout the tumor (**Fig. 4**C). The nuclei are small, oval, and uniform without prominent nucleoli. MSA consistently produces abundant intraluminal basophilic secretions (**Fig. 4**D).

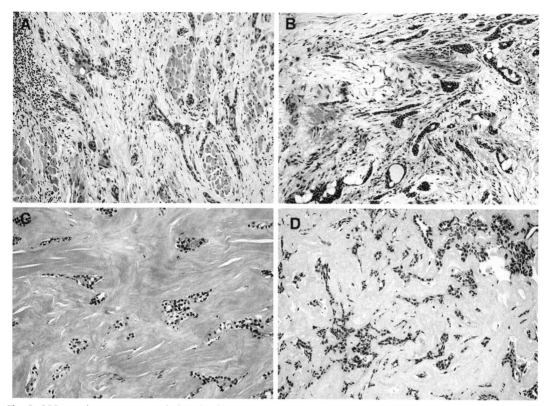

Fig. 3. SCC can demonstrate corded and infiltrative growth that overlaps with SMA, but the presence of focal keratinization and higher grade cytology points to squamous differentiation (*A*, original magnification ×20). The tubular variant of adenoid cystic carcinoma also shows highly infiltrative, biphasic cords and tubules but generally has hyperchromatic, angulated nuclei with at least focal cribriform architecture (*B*, original magnification ×20). Mucoepidermoid carcinoma can also have attenuated eosinophilic tubules embedded in dense collagenous stroma but usually demonstrates prominent goblet cells and mucin production (*C*, original magnification ×20). Although polymorphous adenocarcinoma frequently shows tubular architecture and can have sclerotic stroma, it tends to have more architectural diversity than SMA (*D*, original magnification ×20).

IMMUNOHISTOCHEMISTRY

MSA also has a characteristic immunoprofile that can help distinguish it from most other salivary gland tumors (**Fig. 5**A). Tumor cells consistently demonstrate diffuse positivity for S100 (**Fig. 5**B) and SOX10. They also are positive for p63 (**Fig. 5**C) but negative for its isoform p40 (**Fig. 5**D), a unique discordant immunophenotype that has previously only been reported in PAC.[20] MSA is also negative for mammaglobin, calponin, and SMA.[35]

MOLECULAR TESTING

MSA harbors a recurrent *MEF2C-SS18* fusion that is highly specific for this diagnosis.[35] *SS18*, a member of the SWI/SNF chromatin remodeling complex, is well-known for its role in fusions with *SSX* genes that lead to synovial sarcoma[43,44]; MSA is the first carcinoma to show

recurrent rearrangements in this gene. *MEF2C*, a gene that encodes a transcription factor in the MADS box transcription enhancer factor 2 family, is less commonly implicated in tumorigenesis and has previously only been reported in acute leukemias.[45] Detection of this fusion is performed via either FISH for *SS18* rearrangement or RNA-seq.[46]

DIFFERENTIAL DIAGNOSIS

Several salivary tumors that produce abundant secretions or show microcystic and tubular architecture can enter into the differential diagnosis of MSA. The presence of prominent secretions in MSA raises consideration of secretory carcinoma (SC), which also demonstrates eosinophilic cytoplasm and can have microcystic architecture (**Fig. 6**A) with consistent positivity for S100. However, the tumor cells in SC generally demonstrate

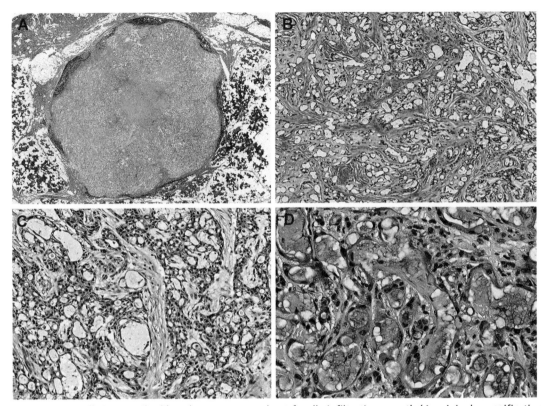

Fig. 4. MSA is well-circumscribed but demonstrates at least focally infiltrative growth (*A*, original magnification ×20). The tumor consists of anastomosing tubules and microcysts embedded in variable amounts of myxohyaline stroma (*B*, original magnification ×20). Tumor cells are bland and contain variable amounts of eosinophilic cytoplasm that is often attenuated in microcystic areas and plump in more sold foci (*C*, original magnification ×20). The lumens contain abundant basophilic secretions (*D*, original magnification ×20).

more abundant, frothy cytoplasm than MSA, and the secretions are predominantly eosinophilic rather than basophilic. Moreover, SC demonstrates concomitant immunohistochemical positivity for mammaglobin and harbors recurrent *ETV6* rearrangements.[13] Another tumor that closely overlaps with MSA is PAC, which not only can show overlapping tubular and microcribriform architecture and myxohyaline stroma (**Fig. 6**B), but also shares its unique immunophenotype including diffuse S100 expression and discordant positivity for p63 and negativity for p40.[20,47,48] But PAC should have less prominent intraluminal secretions than MSA and generally demonstrates more architectural diversity and infiltrative borders, including the characteristic targetoid pattern of perineural invasion. PAC harbors recurrent genetic alterations in *PRKD1, 2,* or *3* that can confirm the diagnosis in challenging cases.[8,9] ACC can also show some morphologic overlap with MSA with a mix of tubular, microcystic, and corded growth and prominent basophilic intraluminal secretions (**Fig.** 6C). Widely

infiltrative borders and at least focally well-developed cribriform architecture help differentiate ACC from MSA. ACC also is a biphasic tumor with concordant p63 and p40 positivity that is restricted to myoepithelial cells; *MYB* and *MYBL1* rearrangements are detected in 50% to 80% of ACC.[37–39] Intraductal carcinoma (IDC) shares an intercalated duct phenotype with MSA, including bland eosinophilic tumor cells, microcystic architecture (**Fig.** 6D), and diffuse S100 positivity. In contrast to MSA, IDC also demonstrates frequent micropapillary and cystic architecture and is consistently confined within an intact myoepithelial cell layer. IDC also harbors recurrent *RET* fusions that can confirm the diagnosis.[10,11] Finally, SMA can also demonstrate microcystic and corded architecture with sclerotic stroma. But SMA demonstrates much lower tumor cellularity with more prominent desmoplastic stroma. Furthermore, SMA is composed of biphasic ductal and myoepithelial cell populations with concordant abluminal p63 and p40 positivity.

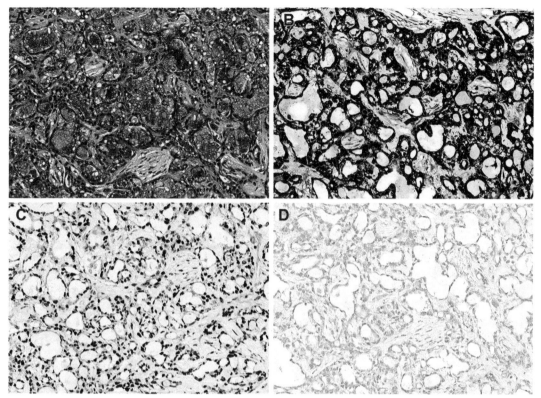

Fig. 5. MSA is composed of a monophasic population of epithelial cells arranged in microcysts and tubules (*A*, original magnification ×20) that are diffusely positive for S100 (*B*, original magnification ×20). They demonstrate discordant positivity for p63 (*C*, original magnification ×20) and negativity for p40 (*D*, original magnification ×20).

SUMMARY

MSA is a newly defined salivary gland tumor that was identified among the heterogeneous adenocarcinoma not otherwise specified category. It is composed of microcysts and tubules lined by flattened to plump eosinophilic cells with bland oval nuclei and abundant basophilic luminal secretions. These tumors also have a variable amount of fibrotic stroma with areas of central sclerosis. MSA demonstrates a unique immunohistochemical profile with expression of S100 and positivity for p63 but negativity for p40. Identification of the characteristic *MEF2C-SS18* fusion can confirm the diagnosis. The uniform microcystic and tubular architecture, monophasic population of eosinophilic cells with attenuated cytoplasm, and prominent basophilic secretions can help differentiate MSA from mimics including SC, PAC, ACC, IDC, and SMA.

SECRETORY MYOEPITHELIAL CARCINOMA

INTRODUCTION

A distinctive subset of myoepithelial carcinoma that demonstrates prominent intracellular mucin production has recently been described under two different names. In 2012, Esteva and colleagues[49] reported one such tumor as mucinous myoepithelioma, a broad category that included benign and malignant myoepithelial neoplasms.[50] Subsequently, Bastaki and colleagues[51] reclassified a larger group of four similar neoplasms that had previously been reported as signet ring adenocarcinomas as SMC because of well-developed myoepithelial differentiation. This review uses the latter terminology to emphasize not only the low-grade malignant nature of these tumors but also their ability to produce serous and mucinous secretions. At least eight additional tumors with a similar morphologic appearance and documented immunohistochemical evidence of myoepithelial differentiation have also been previously reported as signet ring adenocarcinomas.[52,53] These tumors have predominantly been identified at minor salivary sites including the buccal mucosa, palate, maxillary tuberosity, and Warthin duct, although rare cases have also been identified in the parotid gland.[49–53] In limited follow-up, patients have had uniformly

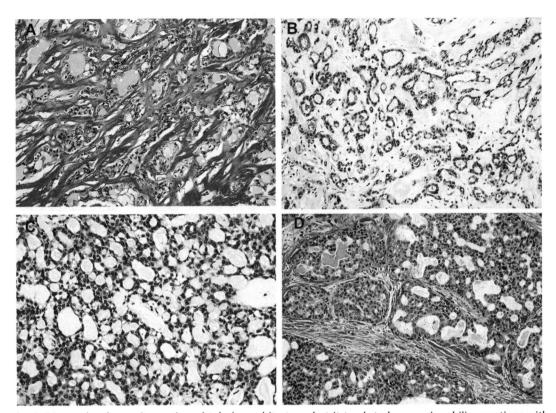

Fig. 6. SC can also show microcystic and tubular architecture, but it tends to have eosinophilic secretions with more abundant vacuolated eosinophilic cytoplasm (*A*, original magnification ×20). PAC can demonstrate tubular growth with an identical immunoprofile to MSA but generally shows more architectural variability and lacks significant luminal secretions (*B*, original magnification ×20). ACC occasionally shows a microcystic growth pattern and abundant basophilic secretions but is biphasic and usually demonstrates at least focal well-developed cribriform architecture (*C*, original magnification ×20). Intraductal carcinoma also shows intercalated-duct differentiation with microcystic architecture but is consistently confined within an intact layer of myoepithelial cells (*D*, original magnification ×20).

good outcomes after complete surgical resection.[49–53]

MICROSCOPIC FEATURES

SMC is composed of sheets, trabeculae, and interconnecting cords of cells with abundant eosinophilic cytoplasm (**Fig.** 7A). Many of the tumor cells contain a single round, eccentric intracytoplasmic mucin vacuole that confers a signet ring appearance (**Fig.** 7B). However, some cases may show similar vacuoles that contain eosinophilic serous secretory material instead (**Fig.** 7C). Plasmacytoid to epithelioid tumor cells that lack secretions are also frequently identifiable. Most cases of SMC have small, uniform, round to oval nuclei with single prominent nucleoli (**Fig.** 7D), although areas of increased pleomorphism can occasionally be seen. Tumor cells are embedded in myxoid to fibrous stroma, with a subset of cases demonstrating pools of abundant extracellular mucin. Although SMC is usually well-circumscribed with a predominantly pushing pattern of invasion, occasional cases demonstrate extensively infiltrative growth with perineural invasion.

IMMUNOHISTOCHEMISTRY

Like all salivary myoepithelial tumors, SMC can demonstrate a variable immunoprofile (**Fig.** 8A). To make the diagnosis of SMC, tumor cells should show positivity for at least one marker of myoepithelial differentiation, such as p63 (**Fig.** 8B), p40, S100 (**Fig.** 8C), smooth muscle actin, or calponin (**Fig.** 8D), although they are rarely positive for all such markers.[50,51] SMC can also show positivity for mammaglobin and Gross cystic disease fluid protein (GCDFP) but is consistently negative for CK20, CDX2, TTF1, synaptophysin,

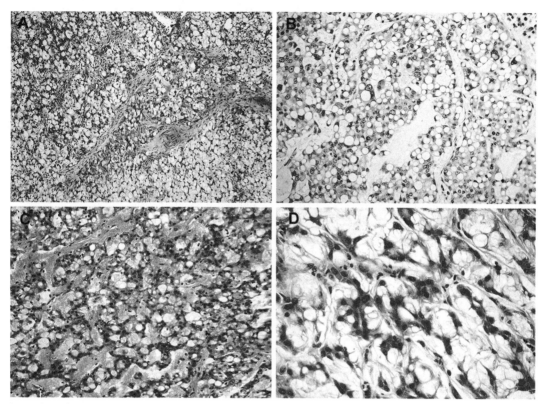

Fig. 7. SMC demonstrates nests and cords of cells with eosinophilic cytoplasm and prominent intracellular mucin vacuoles (*A*, original magnification ×10). Each tumor cell generally has a single eccentric mucin vacuole that confers a signet ring appearance; variable amounts of extracellular mucin also can be present (*B*, original magnification ×20). Some cases of SMC have a mix of eosinophilic serous and mucinous secretions (*C*, original magnification ×20). The tumor cells are generally cytologically bland with monotonous round to oval nuclei and prominent nucleoli (*D*, original magnification ×40).

chromogranin, androgen receptor, estrogen receptor, progesterone receptor, and prostate-specific antigen with retained E-cadherin.[51]

MOLECULAR TESTING

Specific molecular findings have not yet been described in SMC. However, these tumors have been shown to lack the *ETV6* rearrangements diagnostic of SC and the *EWSR1* rearrangements common to soft tissue myoepithelial neoplasms.[51] They also are negative for *ALK* translocations, which are frequently seen in lung adenocarcinomas that demonstrate a signet ring morphology.[51]

DIFFERENTIAL DIAGNOSIS

Although there is no evidence that the clinical behavior or prognosis of SMC differs significantly from other salivary myoepithelial carcinomas, it is essential to recognize this subtype

to facilitate distinction from a broad spectrum of other salivary carcinomas that may not usually be considered in the differential diagnosis of myoepithelial neoplasms. The dominant such diagnostic consideration is SC, which demonstrates overlap with SMC via its prominent secretions (**Fig. 9**A) and positivity for S100 and mammoglobin. SC generally makes more serous than mucinous secretions, has more strikingly multivacuolated cytoplasm, and tends to demonstrate more vesicular chromatin than SMC. Identification of *ETV6* rearrangement can confirm the diagnosis of SC.[13] The microcystic and tubular morphology of MSA can also confer a similar signet ring cell appearance to SMC, and coexpression of S100 and p63 can raise the possibility of myoepithelial differentiation. But the basophilic secretions of MSA are generally extracellular without true intracytoplasmic vacuoles. Identification of the unique *SS18* rearrangement is also helpful in confirming this diagnosis.[35] MEC also can show numerous goblet cells that,

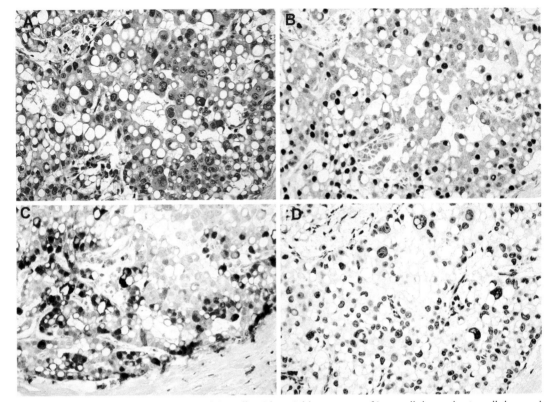

Fig. 8. SMC has cords and nests of eosinophilic cells with variable amounts of intracellular and extracellular mucin (*A*, original magnification ×20). The cells show a myoepithelial phenotype, in this case demonstrating patchy positivity for p40 (*B*, original magnification ×20) and S100 (*C*, original magnification ×20) but negativity for calponin (*D*, original magnification ×20). Although at least one myoepithelial marker should be positive to confirm this diagnosis, expression of individual markers varies by case.

when prominent, may show morphologic overlap with SMC (**Fig. 9**B). However, MEC should also have intermixed intermediate and epidermoid cell populations and, although positive for p63 and p40, should not demonstrate reactivity for other myoepithelial markers. Identification of *MAML2* translocations can confirm a diagnosis of MEC in 50% to 80% of cases.[40–42] Mucinous adenocarcinomas of the salivary glands also frequently show intracellular and extracellular mucin production and even signet ring morphology (**Fig. 9**C) that can overlap with SMC. These tumors tend to show greater architectural diversity, including well-developed glandular, papillary, and colloid architecture, and more marked cytologic atypia than SMC. Although their immunoprofile is somewhat nonspecific, true mucinous adenocarcinomas should lack evidence of myoepithelial differentiation.[54] A final tumor that can show a signet ring appearance with at least focal mucin production is the rhabdoid variant of salivary duct carcinoma

(**Fig. 9**D), another recently described histologic subtype that is thought to be analogous to pleomorphic lobular carcinoma of the breast.[55] However, the rhabdoid variant of salivary duct carcinoma is notable for higher-grade cytology and more infiltrative growth with predominant cords and single cells. It also lacks expression of myoepithelial markers and demonstrates positivity for androgen receptor and loss of E-cadherin.

SUMMARY

SMC is a recently recognized variant of myoepithelial carcinoma that is also called mucinous myoepithelioma. It is composed of sheets, nests, and cords of monotonous cells with abundant eosinophilic cytoplasm and single prominent mucin vacuoles that confer a signet ring appearance. By definition, cases of SMC are positive for at least one immunohistochemical marker of myoepithelial differentiation; they also

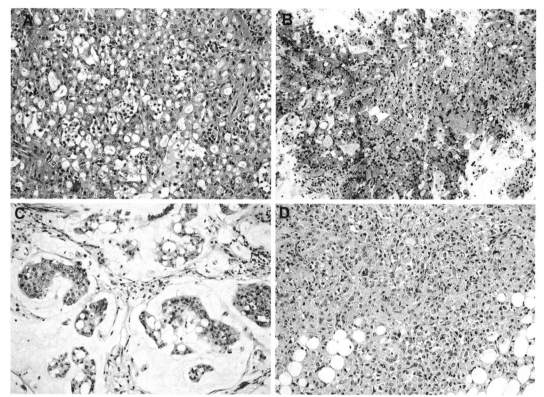

Fig. 9. SC can also demonstrate mucin production and a dense microcystic architecture that mimics signet ring cells but usually also has abundant eosinophilic secretions (*A*, original magnification ×20). MEC can make numerous goblet cells with prominent mucin production but should also show epidermoid and intermediate cell components (*B*, original magnification ×20). Mucinous adenocarcinoma can contain signet ring cells but frequently also has tubular, papillary, or colloid architecture without expression of myoepithelial markers (*C*, original magnification ×20). The rhabdoid variant of salivary duct carcinoma can show focal mucin production and signet ring features but is usually higher grade with infiltrating cords and single cells (*D*, original magnification ×20).

can show focal positivity for mammaglobin and GCDFP. The presence of a single intracellular mucin vacuole, low-grade cytology, and immunohistochemical evidence of myoepithelial differentiation help distinguish SMC from mimics including SC, MSA, MEC, mucinous adenocarcinoma, and the rhabdoid variant of salivary duct carcinoma.

CLINICS CARE POINTS

- SMA is a low-grade salivary gland tumor that is morphologically similar to MAC of the skin with infiltrative tubules and cords embedded in abundant collagenous stroma.

- SMA is composed of a biphasic population of ductal cells that are positive for pancytokeratin and CK7 and myoepithelial cells that are positive for p63, p40, S100, and smooth muscle actin.

- SMA produces scant dense eosinophilic globular secretions that are positive for mucicarmine.

- MSA is a low-grade salivary gland carcinoma recently identified from within the heterogeneous adenocarcinoma not otherwise specified category.

- MSA is predominantly composed of anastomosing microcysts and tubules lined by attenuated eosinophilic cells; it produces prominent basophilic intraluminal secretions and has variable amounts of myxohyaline stroma.

- MSA demonstrates consistent S100 expression, is positive for p63 but negative for p40, and harbors recurrent *MEF2C-SS18* fusions.

- SMC is a recently recognized variant of myoepithelial carcinoma that is also sometimes called mucinous myoepithelioma.

- SMC is composed of nests and cords of monotonous epithelioid to plasmacytoid cells with abundant eosinophilic cytoplasm and single well-defined mucin vacuoles that confer a signet ring appearance.

- SMC should demonstrate positivity for at least one marker of myoepithelial differentiation.

DISCLOSURE

The author has nothing to disclose.

REFERENCES

1. Antonescu CR, Katabi N, Zhang L, et al. EWSR1-ATF1 fusion is a novel and consistent finding in hyalinizing clear-cell carcinoma of salivary gland. Genes Chromosomes Cancer 2011;50(7):559–70.

2. Chiosea SI, Miller M, Seethala RR. HRAS mutations in epithelial-myoepithelial carcinoma. Head Neck Pathol 2014;8(2):146–50.

3. Chiosea SI, Williams L, Griffith CC, et al. Molecular characterization of apocrine salivary duct carcinoma. Am J Surg Pathol 2015;39(6):744–52.

4. El Hallani S, Udager AM, Bell D, et al. Epithelial-myoepithelial carcinoma: frequent morphologic and molecular evidence of preexisting pleomorphic adenoma, common HRAS mutations in PLAG1-intact and HMGA2-intact cases, and occasional TP53, FBXW7, and SMARCB1 alterations in high-grade cases. Am J Surg Pathol 2018;42(1):18–27.

5. Haller F, Bieg M, Will R, et al. Enhancer hijacking activates oncogenic transcription factor NR4A3 in acinic cell carcinomas of the salivary glands. Nat Commun 2019;10(1):368.

6. Jo VY, Sholl LM, Krane JF. Distinctive patterns of CTNNB1 (beta-Catenin) alterations in salivary gland basal cell adenoma and basal cell adenocarcinoma. Am J Surg Pathol 2016;40(8):1143–50.

7. Rito M, Mitani Y, Bell D, et al. Frequent and differential mutations of the CYLD gene in basal cell salivary neoplasms: linkage to tumor development and progression. Mod Pathol 2018;31(7):1064–72.

8. Weinreb I, Piscuoglio S, Martelotto LG, et al. Hotspot activating PRKD1 somatic mutations in polymorphous low-grade adenocarcinomas of the salivary glands. Nat Genet 2014;46(11):1166–9.

9. Weinreb I, Zhang L, Tirunagari LM, et al. Novel PRKD gene rearrangements and variant fusions in cribriform adenocarcinoma of salivary gland origin. Genes Chromosomes Cancer 2014;53(10):845–56.

10. Skalova A, Ptakova N, Santana T, et al. NCOA4-RET and TRIM27-RET are characteristic gene fusions in salivary intraductal carcinoma, including invasive and metastatic tumors: is "intraductal" correct? Am J Surg Pathol 2019;43(10):1303–13.

11. Weinreb I, Bishop JA, Chiosea SI, et al. Recurrent RET gene rearrangements in intraductal carcinomas of salivary gland. Am J Surg Pathol 2018;42(4):442–52.

12. Skalova A, Vanecek T, Martinek P, et al. Molecular profiling of mammary analog secretory carcinoma revealed a subset of tumors harboring a novel ETV6-RET translocation: report of 10 cases. Am J Surg Pathol 2018;42(2):234–46.

13. Skalova A, Vanecek T, Sima R, et al. Mammary analogue secretory carcinoma of salivary glands, containing the ETV6-NTRK3 fusion gene: a hitherto undescribed salivary gland tumor entity. Am J Surg Pathol 2010;34(5):599–608.

14. Bishop JA, Yonescu R, Batista D, et al. Utility of mammaglobin immunohistochemistry as a proxy marker for the ETV6-NTRK3 translocation in the diagnosis of salivary mammary analogue secretory carcinoma. Hum Pathol 2013;44(10):1982–8.

15. Haller F, Skalova A, Ihrler S, et al. Nuclear NR4A3 immunostaining is a specific and sensitive novel marker for acinic cell carcinoma of the salivary glands. Am J Surg Pathol 2019;43(9):1264–72.

16. Hechtman JF, Benayed R, Hyman DM, et al. Pan-Trk immunohistochemistry is an efficient and reliable screen for the detection of NTRK fusions. Am J Surg Pathol 2017;41(11):1547–51.

17. Katabi N, Xu B, Jungbluth AA, et al. PLAG1 immunohistochemistry is a sensitive marker for pleomorphic adenoma: a comparative study with PLAG1 genetic abnormalities. Histopathology 2018;72(2):285–93.

18. Mito JK, Jo VY, Chiosea SI, et al. HMGA2 is a specific immunohistochemical marker for pleomorphic adenoma and carcinoma ex-pleomorphic adenoma. Histopathology 2017;71(4):511–21.

19. Owosho AA, Aguilar CE, Seethala RR. Comparison of p63 and p40 (DeltaNp63) as basal, squamoid, and myoepithelial markers in salivary gland tumors. Appl Immunohistochem Mol Morphol 2016;24(7):501–8.

20. Rooper L, Sharma R, Bishop JA. Polymorphous low grade adenocarcinoma has a consistent p63+/p40-immunophenotype that helps distinguish it from adenoid cystic carcinoma and cellular pleomorphic adenoma. Head Neck Pathol 2015;9(1):79–84.

21. Hsieh MS, Lee YH, Chang YL. SOX10-positive salivary gland tumors: a growing list, including mammary analogue secretory carcinoma of the salivary gland, sialoblastoma, low-grade salivary duct carcinoma, basal cell adenoma/adenocarcinoma, and a subgroup of mucoepidermoid carcinoma. Hum Pathol 2016;56:134–42.

22. Brill LB 2nd, Kanner WA, Fehr A, et al. Analysis of MYB expression and MYB-NFIB gene fusions in adenoid cystic carcinoma and other salivary neoplasms. Mod Pathol 2011;24(9):1169–76.

23. Chenevert J, Duvvuri U, Chiosea S, et al. DOG1: a novel marker of salivary acinar and intercalated duct differentiation. Mod Pathol 2012;25(7): 919–29.

24. Williams L, Thompson LD, Seethala RR, et al. Salivary duct carcinoma: the predominance of apocrine morphology, prevalence of histologic variants, and androgen receptor expression. Am J Surg Pathol 2015;39(5):705–13.

25. Mills AM, Policarpio-Nicholas ML, Agaimy A, et al. Sclerosing microcystic adenocarcinoma of the head and neck mucosa: a neoplasm closely resembling microcystic adnexal carcinoma. Head Neck Pathol 2016;10(4):501–8.

26. Wood A, Conn BI. Sclerosing microcystic adenocarcinoma of the tongue: a report of 2 further cases and review of the literature. Oral Surg Oral Med Oral Pathol Oral Radiol 2018;125(4):e94–102.

27. Zhang R, Cagaanan A, Hafez GR, et al. Sclerosing microcystic adenocarcinoma: report of a rare case and review of literature. Head Neck Pathol 2019; 13(2):215–9.

28. Basile JR, Lin YL. A salivary gland adenocarcinoma mimicking a microcystic adnexal carcinoma. Oral Surg Oral Med Oral Pathol Oral Radiol Endod 2010;109(4):e28–33.

29. Bondi R, Urso C. Syringomatous adenocarcinoma of minor salivary glands. Tumori 1990;76(3):286–9.

30. Ide F, Kikuchi K, Kusama K. Microcystic adnexal (sclerosing sweat duct) carcinoma of intraoral minor salivary gland origin: an extracutaneous adnexal neoplasm? Oral Surg Oral Med Oral Pathol Oral Radiol Endod 2011;112(3):284–6.

31. Ide F, Matsumoto N, Kikuchi K, et al. Microcystic adenocarcinoma: an initially overlooked first proposal of the term. Head Neck Pathol 2019;13(3):487–8.

32. Johnston CA, Toker C. Syringomatous tumors of minor salivary gland origin. Hum Pathol 1982;13(2):182–4.

33. Petersson F, Skogvall I, Elmberger G. Sclerosing sweat duct-like carcinoma of the tongue-a case report and a review of the literature. Am J Dermatopathol 2009;31(7):691–4.

34. Schipper JH, Holecek BU, Sievers KW. A tumour derived from Ebner's glands: microcystic adnexal carcinoma of the tongue. J Laryngol Otol 1995; 109(12):1211–4.

35. Bishop JA, Weinreb I, Swanson D, et al. Microsecretory adenocarcinoma: a novel salivary gland tumor characterized by a recurrent MEF2C-SS18 fusion. Am J Surg Pathol 2019;43(8):1023–32.

36. Chan MP, Plouffe KR, Liu CJ, et al. Next-generation sequencing implicates oncogenic roles for p53 and JAK/STAT signaling in microcystic adnexal carcinomas. Mod Pathol 2019;33(6):1092–103.

37. Brayer KJ, Frerich CA, Kang H, et al. Recurrent fusions in MYB and MYBL1 define a common, transcription factor-driven oncogenic pathway in salivary gland adenoid cystic carcinoma. Cancer Discov 2016;6(2):176–87.

38. Mitani Y, Rao PH, Futreal PA, et al. Novel chromosomal rearrangements and break points at the t(6;9) in salivary adenoid cystic carcinoma: association with MYB-NFIB chimeric fusion, MYB expression, and clinical outcome. Clin Cancer Res 2011; 17(22):7003–14.

39. Persson M, Andren Y, Moskaluk CA, et al. Clinically significant copy number alterations and complex rearrangements of MYB and NFIB in head and neck adenoid cystic carcinoma. Genes Chromosomes Cancer 2012;51(8):805–17.

40. Fehr A, Roser K, Heidorn K, et al. A new type of MAML2 fusion in mucoepidermoid carcinoma. Genes Chromosomes Cancer 2008;47(3):203–6.

41. Tirado Y, Williams MD, Hanna EY, et al. CRTC1/MAML2 fusion transcript in high grade mucoepidermoid carcinomas of salivary and thyroid glands and Warthin's tumors: implications for histogenesis and biologic behavior. Genes Chromosomes Cancer 2007;46(7):708–15.

42. Tonon G, Modi S, Wu L, et al. t(11;19)(q21;p13) translocation in mucoepidermoid carcinoma creates a novel fusion product that disrupts a Notch signaling pathway. Nat Genet 2003;33(2):208–13.

43. Clark J, Rocques PJ, Crew AJ, et al. Identification of novel genes, SYT and SSX, involved in the t(X;18)(p11.2;q11.2) translocation found in human synovial sarcoma. Nat Genet 1994;7(4):502–8.

44. Crew AJ, Clark J, Fisher C, et al. Fusion of SYT to two genes, SSX1 and SSX2, encoding proteins with homology to the Kruppel-associated box in human synovial sarcoma. EMBO J 1995;14(10): 2333–40.

45. Homminga I, Pieters R, Langerak AW, et al. Integrated transcript and genome analyses reveal NKX2-1 and MEF2C as potential oncogenes in T cell acute lymphoblastic leukemia. Cancer Cell 2011;19(4):484–97.

46. Bishop JA, Koduru P, Veremis BM, et al. SS18 Break-Apart Fluorescence In Situ Hybridization is a Practical and Effective Method for Diagnosing Microsecretory Adenocarcinoma of Salivary Glands. Neck Pathol 2021. Epub ahead of print. PMID: 33394377.

47. Darling MR, Schneider JW, Phillips VM. Polymorphous low-grade adenocarcinoma and adenoid cystic carcinoma: a review and comparison of immunohistochemical markers. Oral Oncol 2002; 38(7):641–5.

48. Perez-Ordonez B, Linkov I, Huvos AG. Polymorphous low-grade adenocarcinoma of minor salivary glands: a study of 17 cases with emphasis on cell differentiation. Histopathology 1998;32(6):521–9.

49. Esteva CJ, Slater LJ, Gnepp DR. Mucinous myoepithelioma, a previously unrecognized variant. Mod Pathol 2012;92(Supplement 2):308a.

50. Gnepp DR. Mucinous myoepithelioma, a recently described new myoepithelioma variant. Head Neck Pathol 2013;7(Suppl 1):S85–9.

51. Bastaki JM, Purgina BM, Dacic S, et al. Secretory myoepithelial carcinoma: a histologic and molecular survey and a proposed nomenclature for mucin producing signet ring tumors. Head Neck Pathol 2014; 8(3):250–60.

52. Ghannoum JE, Freedman PD. Signet-ring cell (mucin-producing) adenocarcinomas of minor salivary glands. Am J Surg Pathol 2004;28(1):89–93.

53. Singh M, Khurana N, Wadhwa R, et al. Signet ring carcinoma parotid gland: a case report. Head Neck 2011;33(11):1656–9.

54. Ide F, Mishima K, Tanaka A, et al. Mucinous adenocarcinoma of minor salivary glands: a high-grade malignancy prone to lymph node metastasis. Virchows Arch 2009;454(1):55–60.

55. Kusafuka K, Kawasaki T, Maeda M, et al. Salivary duct carcinoma with rhabdoid features: a salivary counterpart of pleomorphic lobular carcinoma of the breast. Histopathology 2017;70(2):164–73.

Genomic Analysis of Salivary Gland Cancer and Treatment of Salivary Gland Cancers

Doreen Palsgrove, MD[a,1], Sameer Allahabadi, BA[b],
Saad A. Khan, MD[c,*,1]

KEYWORDS

• Salivary gland cancer • Precision medicine • Genomic abnormalities • Targeted therapy

---

Key points

- Salivary gland cancer is a heterogenous group of tumors that presents challenges with both diagnosis and therapy.
- Recent advances in the classification of salivary gland cancers have led to distinct histologic and genomic criteria that successfully differentiate between cancers with similar clinical behavior and appearance.
- Genomic abnormalities have led to the emergence of targeted therapies being used in their therapy with drastic improvements in outcomes as well as reductions in treatment-related toxicity.
- Genomic testing thus aids in optimal classification and diagnosis of the salivary gland malignancy, providing clarity to previously ambiguous and descriptive diagnoses, and in the future may also become the preferred initial therapy.
- Dramatic results seen with molecular targets, such as HER2, TRK, and others, indicate that this approach has the potential to yield even better treatments for the future.

ABSTRACT

Salivary gland cancer is a heterogenous group of tumors that presents challenges with both diagnosis and therapy. Recent advances in the classification of salivary gland cancers have led to distinct histologic and genomic criteria that successfully differentiate between cancers with similar clinical behavior and appearance. Genomic abnormalities have led to the emergence of targeted therapies being used in their therapy with drastic improvements in outcomes as well as reductions in treatment-related toxicity. Dramatic results seen with molecular targets, such as HER2, TRK, and others, indicate that this approach has the potential to yield even better treatments for the future.

OVERVIEW

Salivary gland cancers are rare tumors arising from the head and neck region with varied histology, biologic behavior, treatment recommendations, and genomic alterations. The number of patients diagnosed with salivary gland cancer worldwide is unclear, partially because of difficulty in assessing what constitutes a salivary neoplasm.

---

[a] Department of Pathology, University of Texas Southwestern Medical Center, 5323 Harry Hines Boulevard, Dallas, TX 75390, USA; [b] Texas Christian University, University of North Texas Health Science Center School of Medicine, 3500 Camp Bowie Boulevard, Fort Worth, TX 76107, USA; [c] Stanford Cancer Institute and Stanford University, Stanford, CA, USA
[1] These authors contributed equally to this work.
* Corresponding author. 875 Blake Wilbur Drive, Stanford, CA 94034.
E-mail address: Saad.A.Khan@Stanford.edu

Surgical Pathology 14 (2021) 151–163
https://doi.org/10.1016/j.path.2020.10.001
1875-9181/21/© 2020 Elsevier Inc. All rights reserved.

Estimates range from 0.05 to 2 per 100,000 individuals.[1] They lead to the deaths of more than 2000 people annually in the United States and appear to be increasing in incidence.[2]

Current tumor classification is primarily based on tumor morphology and is often performed in conjunction with supportive ancillary studies, such as immunohistochemistry. As a result of increased availability of genomic abnormality-targeting drugs, there is an increasing role for molecular testing. Diagnostically, many tumors are now considered to be characterized if not defined by certain genomic alterations.[3] Specimens of salivary glands that defy easy histologic classification can also have their diagnosis clarified by a genomic finding that is pathognomonic for a particular salivary gland cancer.

There have been vast improvements in the understanding and characterization of salivary gland tumors. These improvements have largely been a result of the molecular discoveries in various tumor subsets that are increasingly used in clinical practice for diagnosis, prognosis, and therapeutic decision making. Therapeutic options have historically been very limited for salivary gland tumors. There is no drug currently Food and Drug Administration (FDA) approved for use specifically in salivary gland cancers.[4] Traditional cytotoxic chemotherapy has limited efficacy in the published literature,[5,6] and there is a desperate need for additional therapeutic options. The molecular abnormalities identified in specific salivary gland cancer are now being targeted with agents specifically against these genomic alterations. There are increasing reports of outstanding responses to these targeted therapies in salivary gland cancers.

A more accurate diagnosis of the malignancy leads to optimal combination therapy using surgery, radiation, and systemic therapy. Most often when curative intent therapy is no longer an option, molecular drivers of malignancy can be targeted, occasionally yielding spectacular results. The most striking example is often seen in human epidermal growth factor receptor-2 (HER2)-amplified malignancies,[7] although the recent identification of NTRK fusions and salivary gland cancers and accompanying approval for drugs targeting this is an exciting development.[8]

Prior reviews have detailed developments in genomic testing that are augmenting current methods of diagnosis of salivary gland cancers.[9–12] This review describes newer advances in molecular testing that assist in diagnosis but uniquely focus on the new therapies available for some salivary gland cancers with molecular abnormalities. These therapies may eventually become more important for patients at earlier stages of disease but currently are most applicable for those with advanced, treatment-refractory disease. Finally, the authors discuss their current recommendations and clinical practice for managing these patients, which can be challenging, as there are no established guidelines from large national groups.

METHODS

A literature review of English language publications was independently searched using online databases, such as Ovid, MEDLINE, and PubMed, from 1946 to current (by S.A., S.A.K., and H.M.). The search terms include salivary gland cancers AND molecular abnormalities/next generation sequencing/oncogene/targeted therapies/exceptional response/long term survival. More than 500 publications were identified and then further curated to remove duplicates. Studies were included if they discussed treatment options and response, and molecular or gene abnormalities with regards to any form salivary cancer. Any type of study was included in the initial search (ie, case report, review, laboratory research). From there, the publications of greatest clinical significance and rigor were highlighted (by S.A.K. and D.P.). Abstracts were independently analyzed (by S.A., D.P., and S.A.K.) to focus on genetic mutations and their treatment outcomes, genetic sequencing, and current therapeutic standards of salivary gland cancers. In addition, information derived from clinical practice of treatment of salivary gland cancers at the authors' tertiary referral center was used to augment the review of the literature.

HISTOLOGIC CATEGORIZATION OF SALIVARY GLAND MALIGNANCY

WORLD HEALTH ORGANIZATION CLASSIFICATION OF SALIVARY GLAND CANCERS

Salivary gland tumors are one of the most difficult areas of diagnostic pathology, with significant morphologic diversity and overlap between entities. Histologic type is an important predictor of biologic behavior, which in turn influences prognosis and patterns of recurrence and ultimately clinical management. Some tumors are more indolent (eg, clear cell carcinoma) with local and regional recurrence but low nodal and distant metastatic rates, whereas other tumors are clinically aggressive (eg, salivary duct carcinoma) with high rates of nodal metastasis and poor overall survival.[3,13]

The World Health Organization (WHO) still uses histomorphology as the primary basis for classification, emphasizing diagnostic microscopy over sophisticated molecular techniques that are not widely available.[3] There is, however, an emerging paradigm that translocations and gene fusions are common in salivary gland tumors, particularly the monomorphic tumor types. Genomic abnormalities are especially important in 2 entities (mammary analogue): secretory carcinoma and clear cell carcinoma, for which the discovery of specific gene translocations (*ETV6-NTRK3* and *EWSR1-ATF1*, respectively) have supported their recognition as distinct neoplasms and ultimate inclusion in the WHO classification of salivary gland tumors.[3]

EMERGING ROLE OF MOLECULAR DIAGNOSTIC TESTING

Increased utilization of molecular testing has advanced the understanding and recognition of variant morphologies of several established tumor types. For example, ciliated and Warthin-like variants of mucoepidermoid carcinoma (MEC) are newly described variants of a common salivary gland carcinoma that appear to consistently harbor *MAML2* fusions, a finding that is present in most conventional MECs.[14] In addition, carcinoma ex pleomorphic adenoma, which may be morphologically diverse, frequently harbors recurrent *PLAG1* or *HMGA2* gene rearrangements, which it shares with its benign precursor lesion (ie, pleomorphic adenoma).

It should be noted that the use of molecular testing is rarely essential for the diagnosis of salivary tumors. Most tumors can be distinguished by morphology and a judicious immunohistochemical panel. There are even some immunostains that can detect abnormal protein overexpression caused by fusion events, rearrangements, or gene amplification (eg, anti-HER2 for HER2 overexpression caused by *ERBB2* gene amplification in salivary duct carcinoma,[15] anti-pan-Trk for NTRK overexpression caused by gene fusions in secretory carcinoma,[16] and anti-NR4A3 for NR4A3 overexpression caused by recurrent rearrangements [t(4;9)(q13;q31)] in acinic cell carcinoma[17]). Still, many salivary gland tumors share overlapping variant morphologies, and a few undergo high-grade transformation or are late recurrences that lose their characteristic morphologic features. In these scenarios, the presence of a particular molecular alteration can be helpful and even diagnostic.[12] Several notable malignant salivary gland tumor types and their associated molecular abnormalities are summarized in **Table 1**. Unfortunately, the absence of molecular abnormality is not as helpful, because many genomic alterations are not consistently found or there is more than 1 genomic alteration reported within a given tumor type.

There are many technical and cost-associated considerations regarding the implementation of diagnostic molecular testing into clinical practice. With a narrow differential diagnosis, fluorescence in situ hybridization (FISH) is often the most practical and efficient method for detecting common gene rearrangements (see **Table 1**). However, in particularly challenging high-grade cases, next-generation sequencing (NGS) modalities (DNA and/or RNA based), which cover a broader range of genomic abnormalities (eg, rearrangements, point mutations, and copy number changes across multiple genes), may be more useful and/or cost-efficient.

LOCOREGIONAL AND SYSTEMIC THERAPY OPTIONS FOR SALIVARY GLAND CANCERS

From a medical oncology perspective, the specific histologic subtype of salivary gland cancer infrequently changes the therapy recommendations. In clinical practice, most cases present in the locally advanced stage and are treated primarily with surgical resection. Radiation is commonly given postoperatively to reduce recurrence risk. In more common head and neck squamous cell cancer, evidence of positive margins and extranodal extension are poor prognostic factors. In patients who undergo surgical removal of salivary gland cancer, clinicians have no data-based pathologic criteria to select who would benefit from treatment intensification. An ongoing clinical trial (RTOG 1018; NCT01220583) randomizes patients to either adjuvant radiation or radiation + cisplatin–based chemotherapy. Salivary gland histologies that are permitted to enroll in this clinical trial are defined as either high-grade adenocarcinoma, high-grade MEC, salivary duct carcinoma or intermediate-grade adenocarcinoma, or intermediate-grade MEC (NCT01220583). Molecular testing is not required for patients on this study. For patients not participating in this clinical trial, an individualized decision is made as to whether the patient will derive benefit from the addition of any systemic therapy to radiation. In cases whereby the primary tumor is unresectable, it is common to add platinum-based systemic therapy to definitive intent radiation.

Table 1
Molecular abnormalities commonly seen in salivary gland tumor sub-types

Malignant Salivary Gland Tumors	Common Molecular Abnormalities	Other Tumors with the Same or Similar Molecular Abnormality	Adjunct Molecular Testing[a]	Reference(s)
Secretory carcinoma (mammary analogue)	*ETV6-NTRK3* fusion (>95%), *ETV6-RET* fusion (<5%), *ETV6-MET* (rare), *ETV6-X* (rare)	Papillary thyroid carcinoma (subset), lung adenocarcinoma (subset), sinonasal low-grade non-intestinal-type adenocarcinoma (subset)	*ETV6* FISH	3,82–85
Acinic cell carcinoma	t(4;9)(q13;q31) leading to upregulation of *NR4A3*, *HTN3-MSANTD3* fusion (subset), PI3K pathway alterations	None to date	*NR4A3* break-apart FISH	3,86
Adenoid cystic carcinoma	*MYB/MYBL1-NFIB* fusion (majority); PI3K and NOTCH signaling pathway alterations (subset)	Dermal cylindroma (subset)	*MYB* FISH	3
Epithelial-myoepithelial carcinoma (EMC)	*PLAG1* and *HMGA2* rearrangements (EMC ex-PA) *HRAS* mutations in *PLAG1* and *HMGA2* intact cases	Pleomorphic adenoma/myoepithelioma (*PLAG1* and *HMGA2* rearrangements)	Not diagnostically useful or necessary in most cases	87,88
Basal cell adenocarcinoma	*CYLD* alterations (subset), *PIK3CA* alterations (subset)	None to date	Not diagnostically useful or necessary in most cases	3
Mucoepidermoid carcinoma	*CRTC1-MAML2* fusion (majority), *CRTC3-MAML2* fusion (5%), *EWSR1-POU5F1* (rare reports)	Cutaneous clear cell hidradenoma (*CRTC1-MAML2*, *EWSR1-POU5F1*)	*MAML2* FISH	3,89
Polymorphous adenocarcinoma (PAC) and cribriform adenocarcinoma of (minor) salivary gland origin	*PRKD* gene family alterations including rearrangements of *PRKD1/2/3* (PAC) and hotspot *PRKD1* E710D (cribriform adenocarcinoma); *HRAS* mutations	None to date	Not diagnostically useful or necessary in most cases	3

Tumor type	Main gene(s)/alterations	Differential diagnosis	Diagnostic utility	References
Myoepithelial carcinoma (MECA)	*TGFBR3-**PLAG1*** fusion (subset), *FGFR1-**PLAG1*** fusion (MECA ex-PA), ***HMGA2***, and other ***PLAG1*** rearrangements (MECA ex-PA), *EWSR1-ATF1* fusion (subset), *MSN-ALK* fusion (rare)	Pleomorphic adenoma/myoepithelioma (*PLAG1* and *HMGA2* rearrangements); clear cell carcinoma (*EWSR1-ATF1*); anaplastic large cell lymphoma (*MSN-ALK*)	Not diagnostically useful or necessary in most cases	3,90,91
Clear cell carcinoma (hyalinizing)	***EWSR1*-*ATF1*** fusion (>80%), ***EWSR1-CREM*** fusion (subset)	Odontogenic clear cell carcinoma; soft tissue myoepithelial carcinoma	***EWSR1*** FISH	3
Salivary duct carcinoma (SDC)	***ERBB2*** amplification (20%–40%), *AR* copy number gain/splice variants, PI3K/HRAS mutations; for SDC ex-PA: *PLAG1* and *HMGA2* rearrangements, *TP53* mutations, *BRAF* V600E (rare)	Pleomorphic adenoma/myoepithelioma (*PLAG1* and *HMGA2* rearrangements)	Not diagnostically useful or necessary in most cases	3,92,93
Intraductal carcinoma (evolving entity with invasive growth in a subset of cases; also referred to as cribriform cystadenocarcinoma and low-grade salivary duct carcinoma)	*NCOA4-RET* (subset), *TRIM27-**RET*** (subset), *KIAA1217-**RET*** (subset); *TUT1-ETV5* (rare)	Papillary thyroid carcinoma (*NCOA4-RET, KIAA1468-RET*), colon cancer (*NCOA4-RET, TRIM24-RET*)	Not diagnostically useful or necessary in most cases	3,66,94-96
Carcinoma, NOS ex-PA	***PLAG1*** and ***HMGA2*** rearrangements (most); high genetic instability with multiple copy number alterations	Pleomorphic adenoma/myoepithelioma (*PLAG1* and *HMGA2* rearrangements)	Not diagnostically useful in most cases	3

Main gene(s)/gene family are highlighted in bold. Note that this list is not comprehensive and only includes malignant salivary tumors recognized by the 4th edition of the WHO classification of head and neck tumors.[3]

Abbreviations: ex-PA, ex-pleomorphic adenoma; IHC, immunohistochemistry; NOS, not otherwise specified.

[a] NGS modalities (DNA and/or RNA based) may be more useful and/or cost-efficient for certain cases.

It is much more challenging to treat patients who subsequently develop metastatic disease or present with more widespread cancers. There is a lack of well-defined treatment options, and many drugs have been tested and found to have limited efficacy in the setting. Common chemotherapies include paclitaxel,[6] vinorelbine,[18] mitoxantrone,[19] cisplatin,[20] epirubicin,[21] or methotrexate.[22] These chemotherapies all have limited data, indicating their efficacy and response rates are usually less than 10%. In addition, combination chemotherapy using a mixture of cyclophosphamide, doxorubicin, cisplatin, or other variations has been tested and found to have modest activity.[23–27]

TARGETED THERAPY IS ASSOCIATED WITH REPORTED RESPONSES IN HUMANS

HUMAN EPIDERMAL GROWTH FACTOR RECEPTOR-2

Salivary gland neoplasms expressing alterations in the HER2 pathway have been identified. HER2 amplification has been routinely identified as a molecular alteration associated with altered tumor behavior in breast cancer, as well as a predictive of response to HER2 targeting agents. Oncologists have recognized HER2 amplification as an abnormality identified in their patients that can be targeted with monoclonal antibodies against the HER2 receptor, trastuzumab.[28] Newer anti-HER2 monoclonal antibodies, such as pertuzumab, have been combined with trastuzumab and yielded exceptional responses. An example is 1 published report of salivary duct carcinoma patients overexpressing HER2 and treated with a combination of docetaxel chemotherapy as well as pertuzumab and trastuzumab.[29] Both patients achieved a complete response with this combination of chemotherapy and targeted therapy.

Molecular Abnormalities

The most data regarding responses to HER2 targeting agents are with HER2 overexpression or amplification. Using traditional criteria derived from breast cancer, immunohistochemical staining of 3+ is described as "HER2-positive" salivary gland cancer.[30] NGS of salivary gland cancers is useful because it can identify multiple genomic abnormalities from 1 sample.[9] HER2 gene mutations without cooccurring amplifications have been identified and are eligible for clinical trials, such as the National Cancer Institute's MATCH (NCT02465060). However, responses to HER2 mutations are much more variable and often incomplete compared with HER2 amplifications.[4]

Preferred Therapy Options

Large randomized studies are difficult to perform in this population; therefore, the best evidence is in the form of case reports and retrospective series. Although these sources are subject to significant biases, it is reasonable to conclude that a patient with a HER2-amplified tumor should receive HER2 targeting agents. The choice of agent, either trastuzumab[31–36] or pertuzumab,[37,38] and whether to combine it with taxane or platinum-based chemotherapy is an individualized decision. Other case reports suggest a role for Ado-Trastuzumab Emtansine[37,39,40] as yielding responses to HER2-positive cancer, including those that had previously progressed on trastuzumab. The National Comprehensive Cancer Network Head and Neck Cancer[41] guidelines do not specify a particular drug combination over the other, but single or double HER2 targeting agents combined with taxane chemotherapy are commonly used in clinical practice.

NEUROTROPHIC RECEPTOR TYROSINE KINASE FUSION POSITIVE CANCERS

One of the most exciting recent oncologic breakthroughs has been the approval of drugs targeting neurotrophic receptor tyrosine kinase (NTRK) gene fusions.[42] Larotrectinib is a targeted therapy that has been approved by the FDA for any cancer demonstrating NTRK gene fusion. Uniquely, this is not contingent on specific histologic subtype of cancer, or indeed limited only to salivary gland cancers. Many of the patients enrolled on therapeutic clinical trials of larotrectinib (NCT02122913, NCT02637687, and NCT02576431) had salivary gland cancers.[43]

Molecular Abnormalities

Secretory carcinomas of the salivary gland (also known as Mammary Analogue Secretory Carcinoma or MASC) have been identified as harboring NTRK gene fusions.[44] Histologically, these cancers appear similar in appearance to secretory breast carcinomas. Secretory carcinomas are unique in that most of these diagnoses harbor the balanced translocation t(12:15) resulting in the ETV6-NTRK3 gene fusion.[45–48] If this diagnosis is suspected, testing for NTRK fusion should immediately be performed because a positive test will result in specific treatment being selected. Fusions involving TRK and other partners can also be activating, and several have been described.[49] In this evolving field, these activating fusions appear to be responsive to therapy with NTRK targeting drugs. In addition, point mutations involving

TRK are often identified in NGS testing of cancer specimens. In patients who have previously been treated with *NTRK* targeting drugs, these likely represent development of resistance.[50] In patients without prior *NTRK* targeting therapy, the significance of these mutations remains unclear. Although most likely lack clinical significance, it is possible that further molecular characterization may identify some activating mutations.

Preferred Therapy Options

Salivary gland tumors harboring activating fusions involving *NTRK* include most secretory carcinomas. If curative surgery is not possible, the preferred systemic therapy decision is between larotrectinib and entrectinib, which are oral *NTRK* inhibitors. These drugs have a demonstrated track record of delivering responses in patients with *NTRK* fusion-positive salivary gland cancers.[43,51–53] The choice of larotrectinib versus entrectinib is less clear, as both drugs are relatively new and few oncologists have an extensive track record of using either drugs. Novel *HER2* targeting agents, such as the antibody drug conjugate MRG002, are also being tested in salivary gland cancers.[54]

ANDROGEN RECEPTOR TARGETING

Occasionally, androgen receptor–positive tumors are identified in malignant salivary gland cancers. Some subtypes, such as salivary duct carcinoma, appear to have a greater propensity toward androgen receptor positivity.[45,55–57] Androgen receptor positivity has been reported as having prognostic value. Retrospective analyses of salivary gland carcinoma specimens show varying rates of androgen receptor positivity. Those with androgen receptor–positive disease appear to have worse overall and disease-free survival.[58,59] At this time, the prognostic role of androgen receptor and salivary gland carcinoma has not been completely defined.

Molecular Abnormalities

Androgen receptor activity leads to the transcription of multiple genes through DNA binding. It can also lead to increased cell growth differentiation and survival of tumor cells.[60] Blockade of the androgen receptor can be achieved by direct inhibition using antiandrogen therapy. An alternate approach downregulates the gonadotropin-releasing hormone receptor signaling. Both approaches can also be combined for complete androgen blockade.[61]

Preferred Therapies

The overall activity of androgen deprivation therapy using either 1 drug or 2 drugs and metastatic salivary gland cancer appears to be low but has low reported toxicity. To achieve complete androgen deprivation therapy, a combination of leuprolide acetate and bicalutamide can be used. A clinical trial of 36 patient receiving leuprolide and bicalutamide resulted in an objective response rate of 42%. Progression-free survival was a median of 9 months, and overall survival had a median of 31 months.[56,62,63]

RET ALTERATIONS

An exciting new development has been the recognition of *RET* abnormalities being present in assorted cancers, including those arising from the lung and thyroid gland. Rates of *RET* positivity and other cancers are less clear, but there is increasing recognition that fusions involving *RET* are seen in salivary gland cancers.

Molecular Abnormalities

In lung cancer, the most commonly identified right abnormality is a *RET* fusion that results in activation. Conversely, in thyroid cancer, mutations are identified in *RET* that result in downstream activation. In both cases, there is efficacy for the drug selpercatinib, which recently received FDA approval for use in these indications.[64] In some salivary gland cancers, a subset of specimens demonstrates fusions between *RET* and other genes (see **Table 1**). These fusions have been identified in lung cancer.[65] *RET* gene rearrangement has been noted, and intraductal carcinomas of the salivary gland have been identified by FISH. A novel fusion involving *NCOA4–RET* has been identified in carcinomas arising from intraductal carcinoma.[66] This particular fusion is one of the most common seen in thyroid cancer.[67]

Data presented at ASCO 2020 analyzed 59 patients with salivary gland cancers of various stages.[68] *RET* messenger RNA (mRNA) expression was noted in these patients and correlated with outcomes. Of patients, 27% had detectable *RET* mRNA expression in their samples. Patients with detectable *RET* mRNA were reported to have higher time to progression compared with those that did not express it.

Preferred Therapies

Currently, the only FDA-approved agent targeting *RET* is selpercatinib. If a *RET* fusion or mutation is identified and no alternate therapy is available, this drug may be reasonable to attempt based on the clinical scenario.

ADENOID CYSTIC CANCER AS A SPECIAL CASE

An area where identification of any of the above genomic alterations may raise positivity is in adenoid cystic cancers (ACC). Numerous analyses of ACC[69–73] have shown that these cancers rarely if ever demonstrate these abnormalities, making them quite intractable and difficult to treat. In addition, these cancers also demonstrate suboptimal responses to chemotherapy[74,75] and targeted therapies like lenvatinib (a nonspecific targeted therapy used as a multikinase inhibitor).[76] In addition, attempts to treat ACC with immunotherapy have resulted in limited anecdotal efficacy. Moreover, taxanes like paclitaxel appeared to have reduced efficacy in ACC, complicating therapy even further. The lack of therapy options is partially mitigated by an indolent but progressive disease course. A clinical trial using a multikinase inhibitor, lenvatinib, treated patients with recurrent or metastatic ACC. The response rate with lenvatinib was 16%, and median progression-free survival was 17.5 months.[76] Although not a specific targeted therapy, lenvatinib is frequently used in ACC, although additional targets are increasingly being identified in this tumor.

INVESTIGATIONAL APPROACHES

ADENOID CYSTIC CANCER AND NOTCH

Mutations in the NOTCH signaling pathway have been identified as contributing to metastasis of salivary adenoid cystic carcinoma. Immunohistochemical Notch-4 expression is significantly higher in salivary adenoid cystic carcinoma cells that demonstrate metastatic spread and recurrence, compared to the same cancer cells with lower metastatic potential.[77] An analysis of more than a thousand ACC specimens also confirmed that recurrent and metastatic ACC tumors were enriched for alterations in the Notch pathway.[78] Most were in Notch 1, seen in more than a quarter of recurrent or metastatic ACC. Other mutations were identified, including ARID1B and TERT promoter mutations. We now appreciate ACC as not being one monolithic disease and instead may represent distinct molecular subtypes that morphologically resemble each other. A clinical trial for adenoid cystic carcinoma bearing activating NOTCH mutations is ongoing

and may yield a new therapeutic target (NCT03691207).

OTHER INVESTIGATIONAL APPROACHES

Ongoing clinical trials include newer drugs that target some of the pathways that are identified above. Specifically, these include drugs against the androgen receptor, HER2, and NTRK. Another approach is the use of APG 115, which is an orally active MDM-2 protein inhibitor in combination with platinum chemotherapy and wild-type salivary gland cancer (NCT03781986). In addition, combination anti-PD1, nivolumab, and anti-CTL A4, ipilimumab, immunotherapy is also ongoing for recurrent or metastatic salivary gland cancers (NCT03172624). The 2 cohorts include adenoid cystic carcinoma and non-ACC. A phase 1 trial of ADG106, an antibody targeting CD137, has shown some preliminary success in ACC.[79]

Most molecular testing occurs using patient tumor samples as the source. Although tissue NGS is a well-established route of analyzing the genetic makeup of tumors, occasionally there may be insufficient tumor to analyze. In other cancers where molecular testing is of value, tumor biopsies are being supplemented or in some cases replaced with circulating tumor DNA (ctDNA) analysis. In addition, this also benefits the patient in that it may occasionally overcome tumor heterogeneity. A small sampling of salivary gland cancers that have undergone liquid biopsy for ctDNA analysis shows that it may be feasible in those rare cases whereby tissue NGS is not possible.[80]

Many patients with advanced salivary gland cancers have progressive disease that is likely to be fatal; however, molecular testing yields no actionable genomic abnormalities. In these cases, best supportive care or chemotherapy can be attempted. In addition, clinical trials in this population include the use of selinexor a first-line class selective exportin-1 (XP01) inhibitor.[81]

SUMMARY

In this review, the authors have highlighted the abnormalities that are associated with specific neoplasms arising in the salivary gland. Increasing recognition of these molecular abnormalities has led to a realization that these are not merely new entities but in fact had been present in tumor specimens. As the rate of genomic analyses of these tumors increased, these previously unrecognized tumors were then analyzed and accurately diagnosed as these new entities.

ROUTINE GENETIC TESTING IN SALIVARY GLAND CANCERS

Most salivary gland cancers can be accurately diagnosed using established histologic criteria. For these patients, it is unlikely that there would be a benefit to the addition of NGS on molecular testing. Occasionally, focused testing for particular markers may help further establish the diagnosis of a particular subtype of salivary gland cancer, as androgen receptor positivity or *NTRK* in salivary duct carcinoma. For patients whose diagnosis is without question, broad-based molecular testing is unlikely to be helpful and should not routinely be performed, especially if it will not alter treatment decisions.

The authors advocate that salivary gland cancers that contain the modifier "undifferentiated" or "not otherwise specified" should have additional molecular testing performed using an NGS platform. Molecular characterization is especially valuable for those cancers whereby treatment decisions may be altered by a change in diagnosis. The clearest example includes patients who have progressive locally advanced or metastatic disease after prior systemic therapy. In this situation, identification of a molecular abnormality with therapeutic options available may be significantly life prolonging for this patient.

A minority of centers have established testing protocols that perform NGS tests on all cancer specimens at that center. Universal NGS testing provides the additional benefit of discriminating between cancers that appear histologically similar despite possessing unique causes and potentially therapeutic options. It is likely that as cost and availability of NGS platforms make universal testing of cancer more feasible, there may be further subdivisions of salivary gland cancers based on particular molecular abnormalities. It remains to be seen whether the added expense and complexity of global NGS testing on all salivary gland specimens will improve outcomes.

MOLECULAR ABNORMALITIES THAT HAVE ESTABLISHED THERAPEUTIC POTENTIAL

Already for patients with advanced salivary gland cancers, molecular testing can result in drastic improvement in outcomes. Even in highly recalcitrant cancers, such as adenoid cystic carcinoma, the recent identification of NOTCH abnormalities combined with active agent against that target may demonstrate how important molecular testing is. Failing to identify specific subtypes of salivary gland cancer that possess targetable mutations

- Many salivary gland cancers are now defined by specific genomic alterations, which are increasing in number.
- These genomic alterations impact histologic appearance, oncologic behavior, and prognosis.
- For patients with advanced salivary gland cancer, routinely testing for genomic alterations may identify molecular targets that can result in dramatic tumor responses: NTRK, RET, HER2 and androgen receptor.

may perpetuate the vicious cycle of patients not having NGS testing performed, and new drugs not being identified as potential treatments.

CLINICS CARE POINTS

ACKNOWLEDGMENTS

The authors thank Helen Mayo, MLS from the University of Texas Southwestern Medical Center Library for her assistance in literature search.

DISCLOSURE

S.A. Khan received research funding paid to institution by Biodesix, Novartis, Genentech, Merck, Takeda, Bayer, Abbvie, Threshold, Celldex, Bristol-Myers Squibb, Loxo, Gilead Sciences, Pfizer, and Formation Biologics and received consulting fees from Foundation Medicine. The remaining authors have nothing to disclose.

REFERENCES

1. Parkin DM, Whelan SL, Ferlay J, et al. Cancer Incidence in Five Continents Volume VIII. IARC Scientific Publication No. 155.
2. Boukheris H, Curtis RE, Land CE, et al. Incidence of carcinoma of the major salivary glands according to the WHO classification, 1992 to 2006: a population-based study in the United States. Cancer Epidemiol Biomarkers Prev 2009;18:2899–906.
3. El-Naggar AK, Chan JKC, Grandis JR, et al. WHO classification of head and neck tumours. International Agency for Research on Cancer; 2017.
4. Kurzrock R, Bowles DW, Kang H, et al. Targeted therapy for advanced salivary gland carcinoma based on molecular profiling: results from MyPathway, a phase IIa multiple basket study. Ann Oncol 2020;31:412–21.

5. Laurie SA, Ho AL, Fury MG, et al. Systemic therapy in the management of metastatic or locally recurrent adenoid cystic carcinoma of the salivary glands: a systematic review. Lancet Oncol 2011;12:815–24.

6. Gilbert J, Li Y, Pinto HA, et al. Phase II trial of taxol in salivary gland malignancies (E1394): a trial of the Eastern Cooperative Oncology Group. Head Neck 2006;28:197–204.

7. Brown TJ, Sher DJ, Nedzi LA, et al. Cutaneous adnexal adenocarcinoma with exquisite sensitivity to trastuzumab. Head Neck 2017;39:E69–71.

8. Solomon JP, Benayed R, Hechtman JF, et al. Identifying patients with NTRK fusion cancer. Ann Oncol 2019;30:viii16–22.

9. Skalova A, Stenman G, Simpson RHW, et al. The role of molecular testing in the differential diagnosis of salivary gland carcinomas. Am J Surg Pathol 2018; 42:e11–27.

10. Griffith CC, Schmitt AC, Little JL, et al. New developments in salivary gland pathology: clinically useful ancillary testing and new potentially targetable molecular alterations. Arch Pathol Lab Med 2017;141: 381–95.

11. Schvartsman G, Pinto NA, Bell D, et al. Salivary gland tumors: molecular characterization and therapeutic advances for metastatic disease. Head Neck 2019;41:239–47.

12. Todorovic E, Dickson BC, Weinreb I. Salivary gland cancer in the era of routine next-generation sequencing. Head Neck Pathol 2020;14:311–20.

13. Gilbert MR, Sharma A, Schmitt NC, et al. A 20-year review of 75 cases of salivary duct carcinoma. JAMA Otolaryngol Head Neck Surg 2016;142: 489–95.

14. Bishop JA, Cowan ML, Shum CH, et al. MAML2 rearrangements in variant forms of mucoepidermoid carcinoma: ancillary diagnostic testing for the ciliated and warthin-like variants. Am J Surg Pathol 2018;42:130–6.

15. Skalova A, Starek, Kucerova V, et al. Salivary duct carcinoma–a highly aggressive salivary gland tumor with HER-2/neu oncoprotein overexpression. Pathol Res Pract 2001;197:621–6.

16. Bell D, Ferrarotto R, Liang L, et al. Pan-Trk immunohistochemistry reliably identifies ETV6-NTRK3 fusion in secretory carcinoma of the salivary gland. Virchows Arch 2020;476:295–305.

17. Haller F, Skalova A, Ihrler S, et al. Nuclear NR4A3 immunostaining is a specific and sensitive novel marker for acinic cell carcinoma of the salivary glands. Am J Surg Pathol 2019;43:1264–72.

18. Airoldi M, Pedani F, Succo G, et al. Phase II randomized trial comparing vinorelbine versus vinorelbine plus cisplatin in patients with recurrent salivary gland malignancies. Cancer 2001;91:541–7.

19. Verweij J, de Mulder PH, de Graeff A, et al. Phase II study on mitoxantrone in adenoid cystic carcinomas of the head and neck. EORTC Head and Neck Cancer Cooperative Group. Ann Oncol 1996;7:867–9.

20. de Haan LD, De Mulder PH, Vermorken JB, et al. Cisplatin-based chemotherapy in advanced adenoid cystic carcinoma of the head and neck. Head Neck 1992;14:273–7.

21. Vermorken JB, Verweij J, de Mulder PH, et al. Epirubicin in patients with advanced or recurrent adenoid cystic carcinoma of the head and neck: a phase II study of the EORTC head and neck cancer cooperative group. Ann Oncol 1993;4:785–8.

22. Kaplan MJ, Johns ME, Cantrell RW. Chemotherapy for salivary gland cancer. Otolaryngol Head Neck Surg 1986;95:165–70.

23. Dreyfuss AI, Clark JR, Fallon BG, et al. Cyclophosphamide, doxorubicin, and cisplatin combination chemotherapy for advanced carcinomas of salivary gland origin. Cancer 1987;60:2869–72.

24. Alberts DS, Manning MR, Coulthard SW, et al. Adriamycin/cis-platinum/cyclophosphamide combination chemotherapy for advanced carcinoma of the parotid gland. Cancer 1981;47:645–8.

25. Dimery IW, Legha SS, Shirinian M, et al. Fluorouracil, doxorubicin, cyclophosphamide, and cisplatin combination chemotherapy in advanced or recurrent salivary gland carcinoma. J Clin Oncol 1990;8: 1056–62.

26. Nakano K, Sato Y, Sasaki T, et al. Combination chemotherapy of carboplatin and paclitaxel for advanced/metastatic salivary gland carcinoma patients: differences in responses by different pathological diagnoses. Acta Otolaryngol 2016;136: 948–51.

27. Alfieri S, Granata R, Bergamini C, et al. Systemic therapy in metastatic salivary gland carcinomas: a pathology-driven paradigm? Oral Oncol 2017;66: 58–63.

28. Firwana B, Atassi B, Hasan R, et al. Trastuzumab for Her2/neu-positive metastatic salivary gland carcinoma: case report and review of the literature. Avicenna J Med 2012;2:71–3.

29. Park JC, Ma TM, Rooper L, et al. Exceptional responses to pertuzumab, trastuzumab, and docetaxel in human epidermal growth factor receptor-2 high expressing salivary duct carcinomas. Head Neck 2018;40:E100–6.

30. Gajria D, Chandarlapaty S. HER2-amplified breast cancer: mechanisms of trastuzumab resistance and novel targeted therapies. Expert Rev Anticancer Ther 2011;11:263–75.

31. Nabili V, Tan JW, Bhuta S, et al. Salivary duct carcinoma: a clinical and histologic review with implications for trastuzumab therapy. Head Neck 2007;29: 907–12.

32. Haddad R, Colevas AD, Krane JF, et al. Herceptin in patients with advanced or metastatic salivary gland

carcinomas. A phase II study. Oral Oncol 2003;39: 724–7.

33. Takahashi H, Tada Y, Saotome T, et al. Phase II trial of trastuzumab and docetaxel in patients with human epidermal growth factor receptor 2-positive salivary duct carcinoma. J Clin Oncol 2019;37: 125–34.

34. Prat A, Parera M, Reyes V, et al. Successful treatment of pulmonary metastatic salivary ductal carcinoma with trastuzumab-based therapy. Head Neck 2008;30:680–3.

35. Nashed M, Casasola RJ. Biological therapy of salivary duct carcinoma. J Laryngol Otol 2009;123: 250–2.

36. Limaye SA, Posner MR, Krane JF, et al. Trastuzumab for the treatment of salivary duct carcinoma. Oncologist 2013;18:294–300.

37. van Boxtel W, Boon E, Weijs WLJ, et al. Combination of docetaxel, trastuzumab and pertuzumab or treatment with trastuzumab-emtansine for metastatic salivary duct carcinoma. Oral Oncol 2017;72: 198–200.

38. Nami B, Maadi H, Wang Z. Mechanisms underlying the action and synergism of trastuzumab and pertuzumab in targeting HER2-positive breast cancer. Cancers (Basel) 2018;10:342.

39. Correa TS, Matos GDR, Segura M, et al. Second-line treatment of HER2-positive salivary gland tumor: ado-trastuzumab emtansine (T-DM1) after progression on Trastuzumab. Case Rep Oncol 2018;11: 252–7.

40. Jhaveri KL, Wang XV, Makker V, et al. Ado-trastuzumab emtansine (T-DM1) in patients with HER2-amplified tumors excluding breast and gastric/gastroesophageal junction (GEJ) adenocarcinomas: results from the NCI-MATCH trial (EAY131) subprotocol Q. Ann Oncol 2019;30:1821–30.

41. Available at: https://www.nccn.org/professionals/physician_gls/pdf/head-and-neck.pdf. Accessed October 23, 2020.

42. Available at: https://www.fda.gov/drugs/fda-approves-larotrectinib-solid-tumors-ntrk-gene-fusions-0. Accessed October 23, 2020.

43. Hong DS, DuBois SG, Kummar S, et al. Larotrectinib in patients with TRK fusion-positive solid tumours: a pooled analysis of three phase 1/2 clinical trials. Lancet Oncol 2020;21:531–40.

44. Bishop JA. Unmasking MASC: bringing to light the unique morphologic, immunohistochemical and genetic features of the newly recognized mammary analogue secretory carcinoma of salivary glands. Head Neck Pathol 2013;7:35–9.

45. Even C, Baste N, Classe M. New approaches in salivary gland carcinoma. Curr Opin Oncol 2019;31: 169–74.

46. Solomon JP, Hechtman JF. Detection of NTRK fusions: merits and limitations of current diagnostic platforms. Cancer Res 2019;79:3163–8.

47. Marchio C, Scaltriti M, Ladanyi M, et al. ESMO recommendations on the standard methods to detect NTRK fusions in daily practice and clinical research. Ann Oncol 2019;30:1417–27.

48. Skalova A, Vanecek T, Sima R, et al. Mammary analogue secretory carcinoma of salivary glands, containing the ETV6-NTRK3 fusion gene: a hitherto undescribed salivary gland tumor entity. Am J Surg Pathol 2010;34:599–608.

49. Cocco E, Scaltriti M, Drilon A. NTRK fusion-positive cancers and TRK inhibitor therapy. Nat Rev Clin Oncol 2018;15:731–47.

50. Fuse MJ, Okada K, Oh-Hara T, et al. Mechanisms of resistance to NTRK inhibitors and therapeutic strategies in NTRK1-rearranged cancers. Mol Cancer Ther 2017;16:2130–43.

51. Available at: https://www.fda.gov/drugs/resources-information-approved-drugs/fda-approves-entrectinib-ntrk-solid-tumors-and-ros-1-nsclc. Accessed October 23, 2020.

52. Drilon A, Laetsch TW, Kummar S, et al. Efficacy of larotrectinib in TRK fusion-positive cancers in adults and children. N Engl J Med 2018;378:731–9.

53. Doebele RC, Drilon A, Paz-Ares L, et al. Entrectinib in patients with advanced or metastatic NTRK fusion-positive solid tumours: integrated analysis of three phase 1-2 trials. Lancet Oncol 2020;21: 271–82.

54. Li J, Guo Y, Xue J, et al First-in-human phase I study of anti-HER2 ADC MRG002 in patients with relapsed/refractory solid tumors. DOI: 10.1200/JCO.2020.38.15_suppl.TPS1101 Journal of Clinical Oncology 38, no. 15_suppl.

55. Fan CY, Melhem MF, Hosal AS, et al. Expression of androgen receptor, epidermal growth factor receptor, and transforming growth factor alpha in salivary duct carcinoma. Arch Otolaryngol Head Neck Surg 2001;127:1075–9.

56. Fushimi C, Tada Y, Takahashi H, et al. A prospective phase II study of combined androgen blockade in patients with androgen receptor-positive metastatic or locally advanced unresectable salivary gland carcinoma. Ann Oncol 2018;29:979–84.

57. Szewczyk M, Marszalek A, Sygut J, et al. Prognostic markers in salivary gland cancer and their impact on survival. Head Neck 2019;41:3338–47.

58. Masubuchi T, Tada Y, Maruya S, et al. Clinicopathological significance of androgen receptor, HER2, Ki-67 and EGFR expressions in salivary duct carcinoma. Int J Clin Oncol 2015;20:35–44.

59. Nasser SM, Faquin WC, Dayal Y. Expression of androgen, estrogen, and progesterone receptors in salivary gland tumors. Frequent expression of

androgen receptor in a subset of malignant salivary gland tumors. Am J Clin Pathol 2003;119:801–6.

60. Dalin MG, Watson PA, Ho AL, et al. Androgen receptor signaling in salivary gland cancer. Cancers (Basel) 2017;9:17.

61. Gomella LG. Effective testosterone suppression for prostate cancer: is there a best castration therapy? Rev Urol 2009;11:52–60.

62. Boon E, van Boxtel W, Buter J, et al. Androgen deprivation therapy for androgen receptor-positive advanced salivary duct carcinoma: a nationwide case series of 35 patients in The Netherlands. Head Neck 2018;40:605–13.

63. van Boxtel W, Locati LD, van Engen-van Grunsven ACH, et al. Adjuvant androgen deprivation therapy for poor-risk, androgen receptor-positive salivary duct carcinoma. Eur J Cancer 2019;110:62–70.

64. Available at: https://www.fda.gov/drugs/drug-approvals-and-databases/fda-approves-selpercatinib-lung-and-thyroid-cancers-ret-gene-mutations-or-fusions. Accessed October 23, 2020.

65. Bronte G, Ulivi P, Verlicchi A, et al. Targeting RET-rearranged non-small-cell lung cancer: future prospects. Lung Cancer (Auckl) 2019;10:27–36.

66. Weinreb I, Bishop JA, Chiosea SI, et al. Recurrent RET gene rearrangements in intraductal carcinomas of salivary gland. Am J Surg Pathol 2018;42:442–52.

67. Available at: https://www.loxooncology.com/docs/presentations/Drilon_et_al._LOXO-292_ASCO_2018_Presentation_.pdf. Accessed October 23, 2020.

68. Kutukova S, Imyanitov E, Raskin G, et al Prognostic value of HER2, PD-L1 and RET mRNA expression in salivary gland tumor. DOI: 10.1200/JCO.2020.38.15_suppl.e18534 Journal of Clinical Oncology 38, no. 15_suppl.

69. Available at: https://www.redjournal.org/article/S0360-3016(19)34140-9/abstract. Accessed October 23, 2020.

70. Frierson HF Jr, El-Naggar AK, Welsh JB, et al. Large scale molecular analysis identifies genes with altered expression in salivary adenoid cystic carcinoma. Am J Pathol 2002;161:1315–23.

71. Chahal M, Pleasance E, Grewal J, et al. Personalized oncogenomic analysis of metastatic adenoid cystic carcinoma: using whole-genome sequencing to inform clinical decision-making. Cold Spring Harb Mol Case Stud 2018;4:a002626.

72. Frerich CA, Brayer KJ, Painter BM, et al. Transcriptomes define distinct subgroups of salivary gland adenoid cystic carcinoma with different driver mutations and outcomes. Oncotarget 2018;9:7341–58.

73. Rettig EM, Talbot CC Jr, Sausen M, et al. Whole-genome sequencing of salivary gland adenoid cystic carcinoma. Cancer Prev Res (Phila) 2016;9:265–74.

74. Cherifi F, Rambeau A, Johnson A, et al. Systemic treatments of metastatic or locally recurrent adenoid cystic carcinoma of the head and neck, a systematic review. Bull Cancer 2019;106:923–38.

75. Hsieh CE, Lin CY, Lee LY, et al. Adding concurrent chemotherapy to postoperative radiotherapy improves locoregional control but not overall survival in patients with salivary gland adenoid cystic carcinoma-a propensity score matched study. Radiat Oncol 2016;11:47.

76. Tchekmedyian V, Sherman EJ, Dunn L, et al. Phase II study of lenvatinib in patients with progressive, recurrent or metastatic adenoid cystic carcinoma. J Clin Oncol 2019;37:1529–37.

77. Ding LC, She L, Zheng DL, et al. Notch-4 contributes to the metastasis of salivary adenoid cystic carcinoma. Oncol Rep 2010;24:363–8.

78. Ho AS, Ochoa A, Jayakumaran G, et al. Genetic hallmarks of recurrent/metastatic adenoid cystic carcinoma. J Clin Invest 2019;129:4276–89.

79. Zhang L, Zhao H, Ma Y, et al. A phase I, dose-escalation study of ADG106, a fully human anti-CD137 agonistic antibody, in subjects with advanced solid tumors or relapsed/refractory non-Hodgkin lymphoma. J Clin Oncol 2020;38:3105.

80. Okuma HS, Yonemori K, Kojima Y, et al Potentially targetable alterations identified in circulating tumor DNA (ctDNA) from patients (pts) with advanced rare cancers. DOI: 10.1200/JCO.2020.38.15_suppl.e15540 Journal of Clinical Oncology 38, no. 15_suppl.

81. Malone ER, Spreafico A, Weinreb I, et al. Recurrent or metastatic salivary gland tumor (MSGT) patients treated with selinexor, a first in class selective exportin-1 (XPO1) inhibitor. J Clin Oncol 2020;38:6586.

82. Andreasen S, Skalova A, Agaimy A, et al. ETV6 gene rearrangements characterize a morphologically distinct subset of sinonasal low-grade non-intestinal-type adenocarcinoma: a novel translocation-associated carcinoma restricted to the sinonasal tract. Am J Surg Pathol 2017;41:1552–60.

83. Skalova A, Vanecek T, Simpson RH, et al. Mammary analogue secretory carcinoma of salivary glands: molecular analysis of 25 ETV6 gene rearranged tumors with lack of detection of classical ETV6-NTRK3 fusion transcript by standard RT-PCR: report of 4 cases harboring ETV6-X gene fusion. Am J Surg Pathol 2016;40:3–13.

84. Skalova A, Vanecek T, Martinek P, et al. Molecular profiling of mammary analog secretory carcinoma revealed a subset of tumors harboring a novel ETV6-RET translocation: report of 10 cases. Am J Surg Pathol 2018;42:234–46.

85. Xu B, Haroon Al Rasheed MR, Antonescu CR, et al. Pan-Trk immunohistochemistry is a sensitive and specific ancillary tool for diagnosing secretory

carcinoma of the salivary gland and detecting ETV6-NTRK3 fusion. Histopathology 2020;76:375–82.

86. Haller F, Bieg M, Will R, et al. Enhancer hijacking activates oncogenic transcription factor NR4A3 in acinic cell carcinomas of the salivary glands. Nat Commun 2019;10:368.

87. Urano M, Nakaguro M, Yamamoto Y, et al. Diagnostic significance of HRAS mutations in epithelial-myoepithelial carcinomas exhibiting a broad histopathologic spectrum. Am J Surg Pathol 2019;43: 984–94.

88. Grunewald I, Vollbrecht C, Meinrath J, et al. Targeted next generation sequencing of parotid gland cancer uncovers genetic heterogeneity. Oncotarget 2015;6:18224–37.

89. Moller E, Stenman G, Mandahl N, et al. POU5F1, encoding a key regulator of stem cell pluripotency, is fused to EWSR1 in hidradenoma of the skin and mucoepidermoid carcinoma of the salivary glands. J Pathol 2008;215:78–86.

90. Tort F, Pinyol M, Pulford K, et al. Molecular characterization of a new ALK translocation involving moesin (MSN-ALK) in anaplastic large cell lymphoma. Lab Invest 2001;81:419–26.

91. Dalin MG, Katabi N, Persson M, et al. Multi-dimensional genomic analysis of myoepithelial carcinoma identifies prevalent oncogenic gene fusions. Nat Commun 2017;8:1197.

92. Khoo TK, Yu B, Smith JA, et al. Somatic mutations in salivary duct carcinoma and potential therapeutic targets. Oncotarget 2017;8:75893–903.

93. Chiosea SI, Thompson LD, Weinreb I, et al. Subsets of salivary duct carcinoma defined by morphologic evidence of pleomorphic adenoma, PLAG1 or HMGA2 rearrangements, and common genetic alterations. Cancer 2016;122:3136–44.

94. Skalova A, Ptakova N, Santana T, et al. NCOA4-RET and TRIM27-RET are characteristic gene fusions in salivary intraductal carcinoma, including invasive and metastatic tumors: is "intraductal" correct? Am J Surg Pathol 2019;43:1303–13.

95. Staubitz JI, Schad A, Springer E, et al. Novel rearrangements involving the RET gene in papillary thyroid carcinoma. Cancer Genet 2019;230:13–20.

96. Pietrantonio F, Di Nicolantonio F, Schrock AB, et al. RET fusions in a small subset of advanced colorectal cancers at risk of being neglected. Ann Oncol 2018; 29:1394–401.

Printed and bound by CPI Group (UK) Ltd, Croydon, CR0 4YY

03/10/2024

01040371-0016